The Real Language of Food

WITH

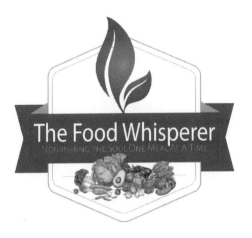

The Food Whisperer

NOURISHING THE SOUL ONE MEAL AT A TIME

Constructive Recipes for a Healthier You

Chef Adrienne Falcone Godsell

The Real Language of Food
with Constructive Recipes for a Healthier You
Chef Adrienne Falcone Godsell

Limit of Liability/Disclaimer of Warranty

The publisher and the author make no representations or warranties with respect to the completeness or accuracy of the contents of this work and specifically disclaim all warranties, including, without limitation, warranties of fitness and eating for a purpose. No warranty may be created or extended by sales or promotional materials. The advice and strategies contained herein may not be suitable for every situation. This work is sold with the understanding that the publisher and author are not engaged in rendering medical, legal, or other professional advice or services. If professional assistance is required, the services of a competent professional person should be sought. Neither the publisher nor the author shall be liable for damages arising herefrom. The fact that an individual, organization, or website is referred to in this work as a citation and/or potential source of further information does not mean that the author or the publisher endorses the information the individual, organization or website may provide or recommendations they/it may make. Furthermore, readers should be aware that Internet websites listed in this work may have changed or disappeared between the time when this work was written and when it is read. The information provided in this book is designed to provide helpful information on the subjects discussed. This book is not meant to be used, nor should it be used, to diagnose or treat any medical condition. For diagnosis or treatment of any medical problem, consult your own physician. The publisher and author are not responsible for any specific health or allergy needs that may require medical supervision and are not liable for any damages or negative consequences from any treatment, action, application or preparation, to any person reading or following the information in this book.

CONTENTS

Black Bean	Red Bean
Split Pea	Thai Green Curry Sans Carrot and Quinoa
Vegetable	Pumpkin White Bean
Chia Water	

Avocado Salsa Sans Tomato	Cilantro Ginger Green Beans

Hummus

White Bean Salad sans Carrot and tomato

Mock Ranch

Cauliflower Tabouli

Cucumber Watercress

Party Slaw

Broccoli, Avocado, Pistachio

Kale Chop

Yellow Squash and Crunchy Sprouts

Zucchini Avocado, Cilantro

Zucchini, Fennel, Tomato Sans Tomato

Vinaigrette

Asian Vinaigrette

Spaghetti Squash w/Spinach

Oven Roasted Veggies

Wilted Greens

Snow Pea, Ginger, Bok Choy

Zucchini, Cilantro Chicken

Rosemary Fish and Asparagus

Chicken Tabouli Sans Tomato

Shrimp and Spinach Sauté

Ginger Chicken with Snow Peas & Shiitake

Shrimp, Squash and Sausage

Beef, Snap Peas & Shiitake Stir Fry

Chopped Steak Tabouli Sans Tomato

Chinese Chicken with Sesame Broccoli

Ginger Lime Chicken

Mediterranean Roasted Fish

Spring Rolls

Creamy Tomato Basil

Thai Green Curry Sans Quinoa

Roast Tomato and Cauliflower Gazpacho

Mango Gazpacho

Spicy Mango ginger

White Gazpacho

Peach Gazpacho

COLD DISHES 107

Avocado Salsa

Zucchini Salad

Lentil salad

Apple Fennel with Lemon

Rainbow Rave

Chard surprise

Grapefruit Salad

Fall Festival

Mango Lotta Flavor

Hot in the City

Summer Refresher

Watermelon Cucumber

Plum, Pepper, Cilantro

Watercress Salad

Ginger, Pear Watercress

Apple Kale

Peach Delight

Fiesta Salad

Summer Slaw

Avocado Something

Kiwi Plum

Jicama Orange

Kale, Berry, Orange

Tropical Chop

HOT DISHES 132

Mediterranean Stir Fry

Asparagus, Zucchini, Tomato

Sweet Potato No Tomato chili

MEAT, FISH AND SEAFOOD 135

Stuffed Zucchini

Kale, Sweet Potato and Sausage Stew

Beef Stuffed Eggplant

Salmon, Potato, Artichoke

Chicken, Spinach, Walnut

Chicken, Roasted Tomato, Artichoke

Zone Fish   Pizza Soup

Grains, Greens and Veggies   Thai Green Curry

Quinoa Surprise   Tabouli, Adrienne Style
Wild Rice and Cranberry   Quinoa, Avocado, Spinach
Quinoa Confetti

Amaranth Stuffed Zucchini   Butternut Quinoa
Mojadara   Veggie Lasagna
Pasta Artichoke   Manchego Mushrooms
Penne, Arugula, Capers, Olives Gingered Basmati Rice
Amaranth Pilaf   Broccoli with Praline Maple
                                Pecans

Shrimp, Feta, Spinach   Zucchini, Feta Chicken
Lemon Olive Chicken with   Quinoa stuffed Acorn Squash
Zucchini
Sausage Pizza Mushroom

NOTE FROM THE AUTHOR

The recipes in this book are a culmination of my efforts to make food that "tastes good AND is good for you." How do I know this? Because of the feedback I have received through the years as to how eating my food has helped people lose those last seven pounds without trying. How their IBS has gone away. How blood pressure and cholesterol have returned to normal numbers.

I have chosen the most simple and effortless recipes as possible, that are not time consuming. I have probably broken every single culinary rule there is and I'm sure some chefs are cringing by the bastardization of recipes and/or techniques that I use. I wanted to take the intimidation factor out of cooking, especially "healthy cooking." In the end, it all comes out tasting and looking good. I feel good knowing that because of the rules I have broken, many people are able eat and enjoy foods they have not been able to eat for a very long time.

Foreward - The Real Language of Food

When asked to write the foreword for *The Real Language of Food,* I enthusiastically agreed to do so. I am not only a fan of Holistic Personal Chef, Adrienne Falcone Godsell, I am a client. I am the last person who likes to cook, but I am the first person who loves to eat delicious healthy food, so I was blessed when my journey toward greater health lead me to Adrienne. I was dealing with health challenges, a hectic work and travel schedule, and feeling worn out. Through working with Adrienne, I was reinvigorated by the foods she prepared and the discussions we had. Adrienne truly cares for the well-being of others and has a great desire to do good in the world.

The Real Language of Food teaches how to discover your healthiest relationship with food, so you can live life optimally. Adrienne poses provocative questions such as, "Do you want to die healthy, or do you want to live sick? Do you want to be enjoying life or do you want the focus to be on which doctor appointment you have next week?"

Adrienne may challenge deep-seated eating habits while encouraging you to expand and take conscious responsibility for your food choices. Through personal life anecdotes and memories, Adrienne shares her journey from growing up being sick and unhealthy to realizing it was up to her to take control of her health. She's a Foodie who has learned ways to love and appreciate food for the wonderful, satisfying, nurturing substance that it is, and how to have fun with it at the same time.

One would think that not having health insurance when you need your gallbladder removed would be a bad thing. But in Adrienne's situation, it was a blessing in disguise. While waiting to afford insurance, she was introduced to the world of natural foods. That lead her to changes in her diet, which in the end, resulted in her being able to get rid of her gallbladder stones naturally and keep her gallbladder.

She does not believe in a cookie-cutter approach. Food has the power to enhance health, concurrently what may be beneficial for one person may not be for another. Adrienne shares knowledge, options, and recipes so you can create a menu that fits your life, today and in the changing years to come.

By changing your relationship with, and attitude about, food, you can change your life. Many of us are not paying attention to the messages our body is giving us when we eat unhealthy foods. The information you will learn in this book may require you to make some changes in the way you eat, yet the benefits will outweigh any perceived sacrifices. Through a process of cleansing your palate with specific food choices, over time you open your taste buds up to a whole new world of flavors, your mind to a whole new connection with your body and your body to a whole new state of health. By focusing on what you can eat during this reset period, rather than what you can't, you will be pleasantly surprised at the delicious and healthy options Adrienne recommends.

After cleansing your palate, the focus shifts to detoxifying your body. During this phase Adrienne teaches you to watch for triggers that cause you to stress eat. Becoming conscious of our patterns is a big step toward making a healthy shift. There are certain foods that will help to detoxify and others that will inhibit the process. A simple but powerful mantra Adrienne shares is, "If it comes from nature, eat it; if it comes from a lab, don't."

Once through the detoxification phase, you begin to add certain foods back into your plan. You learn to feel what foods give you energy, and what foods cause inflammation or a runny nose. You will be more in touch with what your body wants versus what your mind thinks it wants. By outsmarting impulses, you will be eating and feeling much better. You will be developing an eating philosophy that can guide you throughout life.

We have learned over many decades, that poor food choices over time cause dis-ease in the body. Improving how you eat is one of the best health insurance policies you can take out on yourself. Fad diets and quick fix programs may seem like a good idea initially. You may lose some weight and think you are on the road to good health. Often, a year later, you find that you have regained the weight and perhaps more and are less healthy than when you started.

This book gives you information and inspiration to embrace a healthy lifestyle and to enjoy what you are eating at the same time. Gone are the days of flavorless or unappealing health food. The recipes Adrienne shares will excite your senses, and leave both your taste buds and your health barometer satisfied.

Join author Adrienne Falcone Godsell on this journey to wellness. Take simple, yet powerful steps, and reclaim your health!

Dawn Langnes Shear
Chief Development Officer, Upledger Institute
International and Barral Institute International
Consummate Health Foodie

My Story

"It's just baby fat, you'll lose the weight when you get older," my mother said.

Have you heard those words? Did it happen? Did you lose the weight only to gain it back eventually? Let me start by saying, I am Sicilian. I love my Sicilian heritage, but the answer to every problem can't be, "Eat, I love you!"

Birthdays, anniversaries, holidays, Sundays, days off, it didn't matter. We had good food, Mama and Papa made it all. I didn't know what Stove Top Stuffing was when they put it on the table with dinner one night — we called it *Mush Mush*. In the '70s, it wasn't the quality of the food that we had as much as it was the quantity. And we had the quantity; two pounds of pasta for a family of five and no leftovers, for real.

I was a fat kid, 140 lbs. and only 5-feet tall. My parents thought I was beautiful. They told me every day, but at school, I was teased by the other kids. I was called Sister Mary Elephant. Some called me Porky and my sister was called MooMoo — the cow. I got my face shoved in the snow and got embarrassed when it was time for gym or swim lessons; the last one picked for kickball. I came home in tears constantly.

Can you relate?

As I grew in height and became very physically active, the weight dropped off. Still, I ate all the time; just the wrong things. Hot fudge sundaes and French fries for lunch. That's it, nothing else. And after school, when I got to the deli my parents owned, I'd drink iced tea with sugar and maybe a bowl of Papa's tomato sauce with a couple slices of provolone on top – Heaven!!! Then, dinner at home. Now I was just 105lb at 5'5". Should my parents have been concerned? Yes, and we talked about it, but I was eating breakfast, dinner, desserts, subs from the deli for lunch; but not always. I was eating, just not enough for the activity level I was at, and not the best choices.

Then, one morning, I passed out in chorus. Flat out gone—on top of someone in the row in front of me. Of course, the school called my parents, my parents called the doctor, and in I went for a four-hour glucose tolerance test. We knew I would get dizzy if I missed breakfast but what we didn't know until they started taking my blood every half hour for the first two hours (and my passing out even when sitting or lying down) and then once an hour, was that I was hypoglycemic. Things had to change.

It would be so wonderful if there was a magic wand that could be waved to provide everyone with perfect health. You notice I did not say lose weight. I have fought for many years with the whole "weight loss" thing. "Isn't there a simple answer for everyone?"

I'm Sicilian, I want everybody to enjoy food. It was bred into me and I love to help people. I found my calling as having the ability to find ways to get people to eat healthier, and get healthier, while still enjoying their food. The misconception is that healthy foods taste bad and take too long to cook; not to mention they're expensive.

That's not the case.

The direct connection of food and health has deactivated what I'm genetically predisposed to. I'm living proof that food can change your health. By the age of forty-three, my mother had her first heart attack, followed by multiple strokes, high cholesterol, osteopenia and multiple vertebrae fractures. Here I am at fifty with zero prescriptions, strong bones, and a healthy heart. Pills, insulin shots, insulin pumps, insulin monitors — thirty years ago, doctors told you what to eat to get healthy. Now they say eat what you want, but in moderation.

I am sure there are many moments where we do not eat in moderation, not Sicilians and not Americans.

I had a choice/commitment to make and so do you. I gave up "bad"/unhealthy foods. Don't say you can't do it, it's a matter of deciding you want to do it. As a personal chef, I give cooking lessons, dinner parties, and corporate lunch and learns. I feel fabulous when my clients get better and they see the difference it makes.

When anyone loves my food, it's a huge compliment. For me, it's when I can take a conventional recipe, make it dairy free and gluten free and no one knows the difference, I'm a winner and so are my clients.

People say I'm an artist, I'm very creative with my foods. I'm not one to give the perfect presentation on a plate, I'm the one that makes what's on the plate yummy.

Unlike other chefs, I put my ego aside, I'm cooking for you, the client. I want to know what you like and don't like, otherwise I'm doing both of us a dis-service.

I create interactive dinner parties where I bring the recipes and everyone gets to cook them together.

It's so much fun. That's really how the concept of my dinner parties got started. Some people participate, others like to watch as I prepare the food and then serve it.

I have a wine consultant from PRP Wines that comes along and pairs each wine with each dish. Their preservative free, no added sulfite (some vegan, most gluten free), wines are as healthy as the food I prepare.

So, why work with me? Sure, you can cook for yourself... but will you?

You're a busy professional. You are a busy parent. You are caring for your family members, but what about caring for yourself? Shopping for the right foods, prepping every meal, cooking everything to the proper temperature for maximum benefits, timing the meal so everything comes out perfectly and delicious is not easy and it's time consuming. Would you rather do all that or put a few more hours in at work or playing with your kids, relaxing or working on that novel you've been meaning to write? The recipes to follow will take all the pain out of cooking and give you the energy to do all the wants you have on your list.

Living with a healthy eating lifestyle will lead you to finally release that weight and keep it off without eating expensive, tasteless food.

I love what I do because not only am I helping people become healthier through my cooking but I bring people together. Eating is a social activity and should be relished as such. No matter what my eating lifestyle, I'm still Sicilian. Food means fellowship, friendship, and family.

The other benefit of healthy eating, the one near to my heart, is that the right eating lifestyle can help people get off their meds. I received my culinary degree from Johnson and Wales University and was privileged to cook at the Moffitt Cancer Center when they first opened.

I've cooked in Honolulu, Hawaii at one of the top ten restaurants on the island.

My cooking experiences have taken me to Seattle, Washington and Naples, Florida and finally in St. Pete at the beautiful Don Cesar hotel.

I've done every kind of culinary work from working in corporate, private, and franchise restaurants to hotels, and hospitals. You name it, I've cooked it.

I've done everything from hosting to managing and was even GM at the Melting Pot.

Twenty years ago, I fell into natural foods. I began my journey learning about food allergies and veganism (eating no animal product at all, including honey), I had no idea what that was when I was in college.

To be honest, it started out as a way to make money but as I learned more and more about the different needs of people with allergies, especially kids, I was like, "We have to find a way for that little girl to have a cake for her birthday!"

It turned into a passion when I realized that everything I had learned in the hospitality industry and my own personal journey had culminated into having a talent to change or create recipes and make whole foods taste good.

Judy Veal, of Nature's Finest Food, was my assistant back then. She pointed me in the right direction with tofu, Tempeh, dairy free foods, etc. and how to use these as substitutes for people with food allergies. That was twenty years ago and it was hit or miss.

Pam and Moses Brown taught me how vegans should eat. Moses was the CEO of (United Natural Foods). Pam educated people on how to make vegan meals. As much as she didn't like animal products, she knew people were going to eat that way.

"If you're going to be vegan, you have to make sure you're eating right. You need your dark leafy green vegetables with every meal, they are your calcium and iron. Beans are what will give you your iron and B vitamins."

B12 is actually manufactured in your gut so you will not be missing it if you do not eat animal products. Whole grains provide essential nutrients.

So, why am I telling you all this? Why should you read this book?

Lots of people eat things they don't truly enjoy when they believe they not going to be able to eat regular food again due to specialized eating protocols for their health.

I can't let that happen to good people.

I will find a way to hack any recipe and make it good. It'll be up to you to eat it or not.

How you eat can change everything: energy levels, mood, mental clarity, your skin clears up. Sometimes it's not the weight that's lost, but its inches. Your stomach is able to digest what you're eating and you'll rest better.

And that will make me happy. Making people happy is in my blood, just like cooking. It's what I do. Now let's see if we can make food that will make you excited to come back to the table.

Changing Tactics

When you have hypoglycemia, low blood sugar, that doesn't mean you are supposed to take in more sugar to raise your blood sugar level. It means you need to take responsibility to not let it drop to dangerously low levels. As our family doctor put it to me, "If you do not want your pancreas to burn out and become an insulin dependent diabetic, you must eat every 2-3 hours to keep your blood sugar level." My body was meant to be heavier. "The calories going out are not equivalent to the calories going in." Okay, that made sense. At that point, I couldn't tell you where my pancreas was, but I did know I did NOT want to become diabetic. The hypoglycemia revealed why I would get dizzy from not eating and why I would become tired and fatigued. My doctor also told me sugar was my enemy and that I should consider it poison. I needed to be eating five to six small meals a day, complex carbohydrates and protein rich.

I was the only one who could take care of me and I still am. And I needed to learn which foods worked best for ME. What to eat, what I chose to put into my body, exercise, and rest, all of it was up to ME. And, because I was the one who had to make sure I had snacks during the day and eat the right food at lunch and dinner/or four to five small meals a day vs. three larger meals, I no longer passed out, or got dizzy or the shakes, and my sugar was under control. And if I didn't eat every two hours or so? I knew it, and so did anyone around me. Did I like that attention? I think so. Surprisingly enough, even though I was eating more often, and probably taking in more calories, I maintained my weight. I was the sole person responsible for my health. I would have Nutri-Grain cereal with raisins (no sugar in the product at that time, only three ingredients) for breakfast, cheese and crackers for a snack (or a bag of peanuts), salad and soup or a sandwich for lunch, a scoop of tuna at the deli and then whatever Mama made for dinner. I learned how to make cream puffs without sugar (without any sweetener) and unsweetened whipped cream for desserts. I would drink either water or unsweetened iced tea, rarely a diet soda. My parents did not believe in them.

Flash forward to college. A splurge would be frozen yogurt. Why that didn't tweak me I don't know, probably because I had my sugar under control. Once away at college, I did what any good studious college student would do: I ate wings, drank beer, went out dancing and had some cocktails (Long Island Iced Teas), went to parties, and alcoholic beverages were my sugar of choice. It caught up with me because, in the process of having x-rays from a car accident, the doctor noticed I was loaded...LOADED with gallstones, that is. Nineteen-years old with gallstones.

Hmmm. "Did they hurt?" *No.*

"Well, then once your gallbladder acts up, we can remove it," The doctor told me.

"Okay, thanks, Doc." I went on my way.

Until I was twenty-eight, when all of a sudden, I thought my stomach was burning from the inside out. Maybe it had something to do with eating bits of foie gras off the grill while working, or the nightly vodka martinis after work – who knows? But a trip back to the doctor resulted in finding those wonderful gallstones were now begging to come out. Was I obese? No. Did I have a regular menstrual cycle? Yes. Did I eat regularly? Yes, I still followed my semi-hypoglycemic eating with the exception of my adult beverages vs. sugar. So, he wanted to schedule the removal of my unhappy gallbladder. Unfortunately (or fortunately), I did not have insurance at the time so it would have to wait. I learned my triggers, fried and fatty foods, junk food, chocolate, and desserts... and avoided them.

I ate more veggies and prayed for a job that provided health insurance. Which I found, along with a new way of life. That was when I entered the world of Natural Foods as assistant manager in a health food café. My assistant, Judy Veal, shared the neat info that gallstones could be passed naturally (this is not to be taken as medical advice or to be used in place of a physician) and that the gallbladder need not come out, especially since the body needed it for bile salts to break down fat. She told me about a cool product called **Stone Free** by **Planetary Formulas**. I figured I had nothing to lose but gallstones, and two bottles later, my gallstones had dissolved.

It was also during this time that I learned about food allergies and veganism. Now, if someone had told me when I was sixteen, that I would not only be preparing vegan and wheat-free foods, but also eating and enjoying them, I would have laughed myself silly. However, in March 1998, Nature's Finest Foods, Judy Veal, and Pam Brown opened up a whole new world for me and set me on my Green Brick Road to what I am still becoming today. I say "still becoming" because I am still learning and growing.

In today's world, it's just as much the quality as it is the quantity. The food our grandparents or great-grandparents produced and ate is not what we have today. And I truly believe it's why our seniors are having such a difficult time with their health. Their bodies were raised differently. The present generation has it worse because our brains and our bodies are still hard-wired from the caveman days and our food no longer applies. Our bodies have not mutated the way our food has. We are not insects, whose bodies mutate along with whatever it thinks is the latest and greatest way to prolong shelf life, make food taste better (do we really need chemicals to make food taste good?), ship it halfway across the world, stop insects from eating it, and prevent mold and fungus from growing on it.

Our bodies are going to do whatever is natural, normal, or necessary to stay alive. Today's health issues are totally related to what we are putting into it.

What can we do about it?

Take personal responsibility. I don't know if I have the magic formula for YOU. You have to make of it what will work for you. I don't believe in the cookie cutter approach, other than cleansing your metabolic receptors so that your body can function normally — and eventually — naturally. That is why I have options we will be discussing. I do believe that eating should be plant based — by definition, that means 80% plant based on your all of your plates — every day. I also believe a healthy gut is a healthy body. Weak bones? You need trace minerals and Vitamin D (aka vegetables and sunshine). My extra Vitamin D (yes even though I live in sunny Florida) is **Touchstone Essentials** Supergreens +D

Gut issues? You need:

1. Good bacteria in your gut, aka fruits and veggies, and

2. To be producing digestive enzymes to create the acid to break down the food you are eating. My choice is **Enzymedica** Digest Gold.

Liver/kidney issues? Are you drinking water? Not "flavor enhanced" water — WATER. Your body needs water to hydrate the CELLS.

Joint pain, bloating, anxiety attacks, sleep issues? Fish oils/Essential fatty acids are a great choice for everything from inflammation to mood. We lack the good fats in our modern every day eating lifestyle. **Barleans** Fresh Catch Fish Oil is my go-to. Do you have a regular exercise routine? As in five days a week forty to sixty minutes a day, even if it is broken up into two or three segments. I don't hate to say it — exercise has everything to do with your health as well as what you put into your body. Yes, even if you work on your feet all day, your brain and your body need to stay strong through weight resistance and other exercises.

Is it that simple? Or is it that difficult? You tell me. Do you want to die healthy or do you want to live sick? I watched my mother live a slow, painful death. Our minds have everything to do with our state of health, conscious and subconscious. When I'm eighty, I want my kids and grandkids to be discussing what road trip we are taking next, not thinking, "What is she going to be calling about this time?" Heck! I hope they won't find me home because I'm out doing Lord knows what.

My answer to a healthier you is, "Listen to what your body says to you with the food you are eating. Find the healthiest relationship you can have with food and nurture it." I have recipes and anecdotes to assist you along the way. It can be as easy and as fun as you want your journey to be.

As Julia Child would say "Bon Appétit!"

THE PROTOCOL

WIPING THE SLATE CLEAN

Welcome to "Cleansing Your Palate, 101." You noticed I said *palate*. That is because you are still going to be eating during Phase 1. The foods you are going to be eating have been designed to clear your body and your palate of excess. Once your palate is clear, your taste buds are going to be opened up to a whole new world of flavors. They will also be discerning to the yuckies that clog your metabolic receptors. If you listen to your body, it will tell you amazing things that you just have not heard before. Yes, it will be challenging. Isn't that why you are doing this? You are sick and tired of being sick and tired and you know that proper communication between what you are eating and how your body is translating it — is missing in your 'dialect' to take you on your road to better health.

The key in detoxing is to have high fiber, trace mineral and nutrient dense, alkalizing foods that will grab the toxins out of your system and flush them away. The 'alkaline foods' will put your body into a healing state vs. a 'necessary to stay alive' state. This process is made easier when you avoid certain foods that include tomatoes, grains, dairy, soy, fruits, white potatoes, sugars, artificial sweeteners, gluten, and corn. I do believe in a plant-based eating protocol for life. By definition, plant-based eating is 80% plant based. If you choose to go 100% plant based, you may. The recipes in this book provide balanced, nutrient rich plant-based recipes you can live on. The most important principle to remember is that dark leafy green vegetables are to be a daily staple in your lifestyle eating to provide the calcium, iron and B complex that animal product would provide. There are schools of thought/research that say B12 is only available in animal product. That is untrue, because the gut actually manufactures B12, it is a bacterium, so yet again as I believe – a healthy gut is a healthy body! Clear the gut with the extra support it may need. You may need some **Enzymedica** digestive enzymes (***Digest Gold***) and probiotics (***ProBio***, by **Enzymedica** is my go-to) and **Touchstone Essentials'** *Pure Body* to get your gut and entire body in full gear. It is all worth it in the long run.

DETOX

So, you're ready to detoxify your body of toxins via what you are eating. You will have a variety of experiences during this time ranging from hunger pangs to finding your stressors that cause you to eat (commonly known as "stress eating") to getting upset when the person next to you is chewing too loudly. There is a food protocol to follow as you journey down the detox path. There are certain foods that assist your cleanse and there are foods that inhibit the process. We are putting your body into a healing state by eating foods that are more alkaline and low acid foods. You will also notice most of my recipes are plant based. That is because most people know how to prepare meat/fish/seafood, but they do not know how/find it too time consuming to prepare plant-based dishes. It has been my experience that the demand for plant-based dishes to complement the rest of one's plate is where the demand is. For those that want to be 100% plant based, there are recipes with beans. For those that want to be adding the 80% plan based to their meat/fish/seafood – here is your answer. During the first ten to fourteen days, your body will probably 'crave' the more acidic foods — i.e.: sugar, coffee, chocolate, bread. You will play with this 4 -6 weeks. Please note, I do not use meat or cheese substitutes in any of my recipes, only beans, seeds and nuts. I do not believe a manufactured meat/dairy substitute does you or your body any justice. If there is a product you prefer to use, you may. I simply do believe if it comes from nature, eat it, if it comes from a lab, don't.

The no list:

> yeast, sugar, tomatoes, vinegar, all grains containing gluten - wheat, oats, rye, barley, spelt, kamut, all gluten free grains as well – rice, amaranth, quinoa, brown rice, buckwheat, honey, dairy (including dairy yogurt), chocolate, artificial sweeteners, fruit (except for those on the 'yes list'), corn, potatoes, fruit juices, coffee.

The yes list (although there are 'cheats' (c) on here that can aggravate):

> all green veggies, sweet potatoes (c), fresh lemon, blueberries, raspberries, blackberries, nuts, seeds, carob, stevia, xylitol(c), raw carrot occasionally, squash (any type), egg, raw apple cider vinegar, raw agave nectar(c), beans, Rice Dream rice milk, Almond Dream unsweetened milk, Coconut Bliss ice cream(c), raw cocoa nibs, yerba mate tea.

You will notice there are not any grains in the recipes provided during the detox stage, even gluten free grains. That is because there is a train of thought that grains inhibit metabolic (and brain) processes as well. You can look at the research in *Dr. Perlmutter's* book ***"Grain Brain: The Surprising Truths about Wheat, Carbs and Sugars, Your Brain's Silent Killers."*** I have played around with this theory/research and have found it to be beneficial at certain points in my life. I believe, since our bodies are made up of an average of 65% water, according to Guyton, Arthur C. (1991). *Textbook of Medical Physiology* (8th ed.), that there is not a *one size fits all* eating lifestyle. Our body's nutritional needs, as well as our taste buds, change...shift. The needs and nutritional demands of the body morph and grow as our lives do. Therefore, when we notice the skin on our face getting red (rosacea ?) or bloating and gas after we have grains (gluten and also gluten free), eliminate the foods in this part of the protocol and see what results you yield.

Basically protein, green veggies, beans, seeds, nuts and a few sweet potatoes. And even then, you may need to pull beans and sweet potatoes out as well as the other night shades – eggplant, tobacco and peppers. High fiber is very important, thirty-five to forty grams a day. This is to cleanse the toxins out of your system once they are shaken up and running around. Water, at least half your body weight in ounces of water.

Did you know according to the same research in **Guyton, Arthur C**. (1991). *Textbook of Medical Physiology* (8th ed.) "The body water constitutes as much as 75% of the body weight of a newborn infant, whereas some obese people are as little as 45% water by weight."? For me, that means that either we gain weight when we are not eating nutritionally sound food as well as not drinking enough water, or we stay obese because we are nutritionally deficient and not drinking enough water as well. No, tea is not counted as water. You may have that in addition to your water, but it is not counted as your water intake. Add freshly-squeezed lemon to your water if you do not like the taste of it. Water is essential for flushing the toxins out of your system. Yes, you will be emptying your bladder frequently, but you are supposed to. We are not supposed to keep garbage in our bodies, just like we are not supposed to keep garbage in our homes. We have out body for our whole lives, let's keep it as healthy as we are able to.

The other process taking place during the Detox Phase is to find, identify and write down/journal what I like to call "your stress eating triggers". I can say I am a stress eater. To enhance my detox process, I use **Touchstone Essentials Pure Body** and **Super Greens +D** every day. It is the only gentle daily detox I know that does not strip the body of essential nutrients. **Pure Body** is the zeolite Clinoptilolite, which naturally draws negatively charged ions to it (heavy metals, chemical and environmental toxins). With the way that **Touchstone Essentials** cleans and processes this zeolite, it is in and out of your body in forty-three hours, without stripping the essential nutrients out of your organs. Plus, once you rid your body of toxins you want to replace those empty areas with nutrition, which is why the **Supergreens + D** is so great. Plant-based calcium, iron, and Vitamin D fits right into my lifestyle of what comes from the ground, my body knows what to do with it. I get the clarity of what my body is begging for vs. *what my mind **thinks** it **wants**.* That is why I use the title **The Real Language of Food**. It is time to start listening to what our body is begging for, to understand the dialect of each food and how our body can use (or not) it to heal itself. Salty cravings are typically the body's need for natural sources of potassium and sodium. Please note the use of the word ***natural***. So that means cucumbers, celery, zucchini, nuts, seeds, sprouted beans. Sweet cravings go into natural sugars, but also the body's need for serotonin, which is produced primarily in the gut, which is primarily what is congested and needs to be cleansed and cleared. Fatty food cravings have to do with not getting enough of the right fats. As in seeds and nuts. Not chips and nachos. We are not meant to be consuming fried foods on a daily basis. That is one reason we are so malnourished in today's world. We are stuffing ourselves full of processed foods and then our bodies are still craving the nourishment it needs to survive. It robs calcium from our bones to reduce the acid in our body. The brain creates more cholesterol when we are told there is too much in it and are taking medication that blocks it. Then we wonder why there is dementia and sexual issues. In the book ***The Power of Habit***, by *Charles Duhigg*, he discusses the fact that the key to creating a new habit is by identifying the trigger, **changing the response** and retaining the reward. Think about this – can you stop rush hour traffic? No, but you can change your response to it. And still feel relieved afterwards. Can you change your child/teenager from having a meltdown over a punishment? I haven't found a way yet, but please let me know if you do. No, but your response can change from eating chocolate, having a cocktail (or three), consuming an entire bag of chips to refrain from arguing with him/her. And still get the peace after the waters have settled. I am not an authority on behavior and psychology. I am a foodie who has learned ways to love and appreciate food for the wonderful, satisfying, nurturing, energizing, flavorful substance that it is and how to appreciate it without demonizing it.

A mental health practitioner I worked with once said during a meditation, "What are you trying to stuff back down into yourself when you are stress eating?" Journal it. Talk with a friend. Talk with a professional. Exercise. Meditate. I notice myself sometimes rummaging through the kitchen when I am not 'hungry.' I am needing to talk about something, but instead I find myself searching for a way to stuff it back down. So, I make sure not to keep anything that I would use as a pacifier in my kitchen and journal or exercise if whoever I need to talk with is not there. And it is good to journal so when the time comes to discuss that topic, I have worked out a calm way vs. a very raw way of conversing.

What have you got to lose by avoiding these foods other than excess weight, bad skin, poor digestion, joint aches, chronic inflammation, sugar, blood pressure, and cholesterol issues?

THE VOCABULARY

How, What, When, Why, and Where You Eat Makes Your Health What it Is.

After the Detox section, over the next three weeks, you will slowly begin to add foods back into your eating lifestyle. This is to slowly reintroduce what I like to call the food antagonists back into your body and see what works (digests) and what doesn't. I do not think restricting healthy carbs in your body helps it function naturally. All foods that come from the earth are here for a reason. Call it **The Cheat System Diet (Jackie Wicks), Stress Less Living (Thea Singer)**, the **Sonoma (Dr. Connie Gutterson), Virgin Diet (JJ Virgin), South Beach (Arthur Agatston. M.D.), Paleo (Loren Cordain Ph.D.), Eat Right 4 Your Blood Type (Peter J D'Adamo), The Zone (Barry Sears Ph.D.), Perricone (Nicholas Perrocone M.D.), The Whole 30 (Melissa Hartwig/ Dallas Hartwig)**: all these eating lifestyles have some things in common with this lifestyle – no processed foods, no artificial sweeteners, fresh fruits and veggies in abundance, education about foods and their effects on the body's metabolic functioning, food antagonists (allergens), enhancing digestion and, therefore, encouraging enhanced metabolic energy and vitality through having your body work on a natural level vs. normal or necessary level.

You are only as healthy as you permit yourself to be. The body self regulates. What does that mean? Simply put, what goes in is what comes out. Or doesn't. And sits, festers, ferments, mutates, and becomes something we do not want it to become somewhere in our body. Whether we are talking physical ingestion and digestion of food and the excretion of the waste, or whether we're talking about the energy we receive (or not) from what we ingest. Did you know that we can use up to 80% of our energy just in digesting food once we eat? Elkaim, Yuri, "Health Benefits of Fasting." Eating for Energy Blog. Yuri Elkaim, 22 Oct 2009. Web. 2 Aug 2010. So, by cleansing our metabolic receptors with the food we are eating and using digestive enzymes (**Digest Gold** is my go-to by **Enzymedica**) not only are we giving our bodies a fresh opportunity to work properly, but also our brain will clearly translate what our bodies are asking for - nutrient dense foods vs. a quick fix. And when I added **Touchstone Essentials Pure Body and Supergreens+D** into the mix, my metabolic receptors are in a continual state of sloughing off layers (and years) of toxins from my system.

The Vocabulary is the second step in resetting your body. Now that you have a clean palate and plate, you will begin to reintroduce foods back into your system with the intention of recognizing triggers that maybe cause inflammation, bloating, a runny nose. Some foods may give you more energy, some may leave you lacking. The point is that by giving yourself a clear slate, **you** get to make your own rules because **you** will be **more in touch with what your body and the food you are eating is telling you**. One set of rules I like to follow is this:

1. All fruits before noon. Fruits have bulk to them, along with water. Let these be your beginning of the day

foods to get your system 'flowing.' Besides that, you don't want your fruit "fermenting" on top of whatever else you will eat during the course of the day, bubbling and boiling, causing gas and bloating issues.

2. Finish eating your carbs, all of them, by 4pm. This seems to be a golden rule that personal trainers swear by for their clients, and I have to agree. After playing around with this, look at the logistics – your activity levels are far higher in the morning and afternoon than they are in the evening. You need your complex carbs for energy. Why have them at night when they can sit and turn into fat vs. being used as energy for the body and burn the fat?

3. No food after 7pm. Seriously, this can be difficult, but unless you have the life of a Sumo wrestler, where are all those calories going to be used if you are eating at 8pm and going to bed at 11pm? You are not going to tell me that you are going to work out at 9pm after you have worked all day, are you? One of my favorite clients, when I worked in health food cafes, and I would joke around some afternoons about "calorie deficit.' This is when you have been 'too busy' to eat breakfast, only a snack bar for lunch and get around to eating at 3pm. You are STARVING! So then you begin to eat. And you really cannot curb that hunger and, so continue eating, until maybe 9pm. Why? Because you have gone all day without eating, being active without giving your body any fuel to continue with your day. And so what does your body use for fuel? Your OWN MUSCLE! No, it's not using that store of fat you have on your thighs, waist, arms, and belly. That is what is being created due to your brain thinking it is going into a famine and protecting all

your organs. Get those calories in when your body needs them. You are doing a great disservice to your body by not eating regularly.

During **The Vocabulary**, you also get to put into action the great lessons you learned during the Detox Phase of interpreting your cravings. The 4-6 weeks that you put into acknowledging, and addressing stress eating and finding creative ways to avoid the sweet/salty tooth still needs to become a habit. You now should be comprehending the difference between "I am stressed and need to calm down" and "I am stressed, give me something sweet/salty to continue to run away from the Saber-tooth tiger." Our brains are still hardwired to prehistoric days. Unfortunately, social media has capitalized on this with its various promotions. It is up to us to be adults, soothe the inner child in us without hurting him/her. We need to use our words to tell the inner child, "Yes, it would be nice to have a piece of chocolate right now, but if you are going to demand five pieces because they are the fun sized, and you deserve them for all the work you have done, I have to say NO." You are borderline diabetic, you are fifteen pounds overweight and you haven't worked out regularly in three weeks? Once you are back on track with all your goals, we'll have that chocolate. What do you have to lose by enhancing your health? No more medications. A full night's sleep. More energy throughout the entire day. Your skinny clothes getting too big. Enjoying a few bits of that cake and saying, "That was really good, but it's not as good as I remember." Most of what we **think** tastes good, feels **awful** twenty minutes later. Instant gratification is what has you at the health crisis you are right now Learning **The Real Language of Food** is what will get you to a healthier place where you can and will enjoy everything in moderation, by choice.

PYGMALION

Well, you have made it. After four to six weeks of cleansing and 3 weeks learning the vocabulary for **The Real Language of Food**, you may now take on the full conversation food has to offer. Now you will reintroduce grains, (meat, fish) and dairy, if you so choose. By keeping all the commonly known food antagonists out of your system, you may have felt freer, lighter, more energized. Some people's bodies only need to be reset, others may find their lives are not lacking anything by not having these food items in their daily eating. It is very easy to stay on a plant-based (vegan) protocol without lacking any vitamin or minerals. In fact, the body gets more calcium out of dark leafy green vegetables and sesame seeds than it does from dairy, since it is pasteurized anyhow. You are being reintroduced into the world of food for what it is with a whole new perspective. Just like Eliza Doolittle in *Pygmalion* (or *My Fair Lady*), was taught the proper way to listen, hear and speak her proper language, it was then left up to her to use it in her everyday life. And she was lost at first. "Where am I to go, what am I to do with myself now that you have made me a lady?' she asked Henry Higgins. I am asking you the same question. What are you going to do now that you have been equipped with **The Real Language of Food**? I have armed you enough recipes, knowledge and decision-making skills to send you off into the real world. I hope you read the books I have recommended. I am not a know-it-all, and it is in knowing there are like-minded professionals that I want to share what I have learned. You are an individual.

You did not come from a one-size-fits-all. You have to see what works for you. And as the seasons change, and life changes, and your needs change, so will how you eat. That doesn't mean you have to fall back into something that will make you sick. To me, it is about living a quality life until the end. Food, especially today's food, has so much to do with our health. What, why, when, where, and how we eat makes all the difference in our health. Learn how to *interpret* what your mind *thinks* your body is craving and learn each food's dialect with your body. Foods needed by the body change just like seasons do.

E-CISE

Surely you have been thinking that any eating protocol would be complete if there was some sort of exercise/strengthening support, right?

So, 4 years ago, I read *Jackie Wicks'* book *The Cheat System Diet*, because as every good Holistic Personal Chef does, they read all the newest eating protocols on the market to be up to date on client requests. In *The Cheat System*, *Jackie Wicks* has a progressive protocol of 'stretches' to strengthen the core while following her protocol. The creator of said protocol is founder of *Pain Free Living* **Pete Egoscue**. Little did I know that I would not only be sold on **Egoscue E-cises**, but also become a number one fan in the Tampa Bay area. Through following the E-cise course work, I did notice my core becoming stronger, my digestion getting more enhanced (healthy gut muscles healthy body). A few months later I was at a networking meeting and met the Director of the then newest Egoscue Clinic right here in Tampa! Michelle went on to speak about the clinic and *Pain Free Living* and the Grand Opening happening within the next week. I did not catch the name of the clinic until she passed cards around (I was caught up in the energy of the moment) and when I saw **Egoscue** I exclaimed "I know **Egoscue**!!!! I have been playing around with *The Cheat System* protocol for the past month!!" I had the privilege of meeting **Pete Egoscue** at the open house and became colleagues with Michelle and **The Egoscue Method. The Egoscue Method** (you can have one on one therapy, even if you do not live near a clinic) not only got my right arm back in communication with the rest of my body (I had been in a car accident 4 years prior and with a TBI that still had residual numbness in my right arm on occasion) but also corrected TMJ I had acquired from a car accident 25 years prior. Anyone who has TMJ, knows what a miracle that is. Pete and Brian Bradley have put together a **Real Language of Food** protocol to enhance the results you may achieve playing around with **The Real Language of Food recipes**. Try it, you'll like it. Maybe even want to delve further into The Egoscue Method for enhanced postural alignment, up your exercise game (I cut 3 minutes off my jogging time as well with **Egoscue**) or rid your life of pain.

A Note From Brian Bradley

Vice President, Brand Development and Special Programs

Here's another note to ponder about Egoscue. Not only do the Egoscue therapists focus on the true cause of your chronic pain symptoms by going after the root of the pathological movement, but a side effect of this is an increase in the functional efficiency of the lymphatic system.

When you do your Egoscue menu and change your upper back position, you become more Hip Driven. This efficient movement allows the pumps in the ankles, knees, hips and shoulders to do their job and move fluid efficiently through your system.

One way to know that your body is out of alignment is by closing your eyes and finding out where your balance is daily. With your eyes closed ask yourself these questions.

Is the weight even from left to right on each foot? Is the weight in each foot centered in the ball of the foot or is there more weight in the heel of one foot and the ball of the other, possibly showing you that there is rotation in the rest of the body... making compensations for your posture dysfunction.

When you feel that your body is out of balance, be sure to re-check it after you do your exercises because you'll be amazed at how quickly your body responds and becomes more functional.

The remedy? Do your Egoscue as your foundation to start your day!

If you have any specific questions, email Egoscue at painfree@egoscue.com

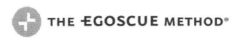

E-Cises

These E-cises have been created to do in order to create maximum postural alignment in your body – aka strong core muscles. You have 2 groups to work out with alternating Monday, Wednesday, Friday and Tuesday, Thursday, Saturday. The 10 minutes that it takes will make you a very happy (healthy and stronger) person. It's your body, you have decided to commit to being a healthier you, why would you choose to let your muscles miss out on this new commitment? You will be receiving a cumulative effect going into the weeks, months and years ahead doing these.

You will my also go to Egoscue.com in case you would like a personal protocol for Pain free Living or to enhance your athletic performance. Check out locations and see if there is an Egoscue Clinic near you!

Monday - Wednesday - Friday

Standing Arm Circles

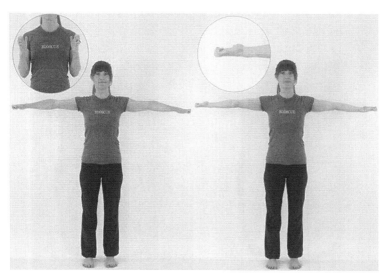

Sets = 2, Reps = 40

How to Perform

1. Stand facing mirror with your feet pointed straight ahead. Place your finger tips into the pad of each hand and point your thumb straight out.

2. This hand position is imperative to the exercise being done correctly. It is called the "golfer's grip".

3. Squeeze your shoulder blades together backwards and bring your arms out to your sides at shoulder level.

4. With your palms facing downward, circle up and

forward for the repetitions specified. With your palms facing upward, circle up and back for the desired repetitions.

5. Remember to keep your feet straight and your shoulder blades squeezed together.

Fun Facts

This exercise promotes bilateral lumbar function through thoracic stabilization.

Standing Elbow Curls

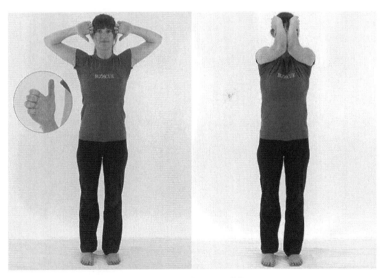

Sets = 1, Reps = 25

How to Perform

1. Stand against a wall with your feet pointed straight ahead.

2. Keep your heels, hips, upper back and head against the wall.

3. Place your knuckles against your temples with your thumbs pointed down to your shoulders.

4. Open your elbows so that they are against the wall and close your elbows together in front of your face.

5. REPEAT

Fun Facts

This exercise promotes proper positioning of all load joints while performing thoracic flexion and extension.

Standing Overhead Extension

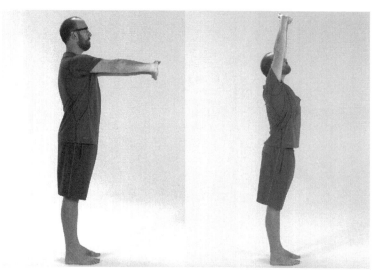

Sets = 1, Reps = 1, Duration = 00:01:00

How to Perform

1. Stand with your feet pointing straight and hip width apart.

2. Interlace your fingers together and reach your arms overhead, pressing your hands to the ceiling with palms up.

3. Look up toward your hands and keep your arms straight, do not bend at the elbow. Do not lean back.

4. Try to keep your arms directly overhead, not forward of your head. Relax your stomach muscles.

5. Hold as directed on your menu.

Fun Facts

This exercise promotes lumbar and thoracic extension through bilateral hip demand.

Tuesday - Thursday - Saturday

Standing Overhead Extension

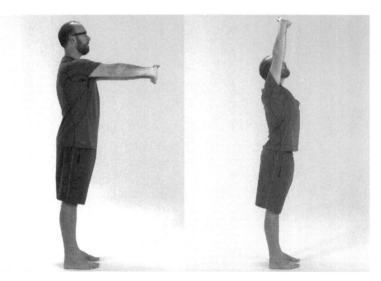

Sets = 1, Reps = 1, Duration = 00:01:00

How to Perform

1. Stand with your feet pointing straight and hip width apart.

2. Interlace your fingers together and reach your arms overhead, pressing your hands to the ceiling with palms up.

3. Look up toward your hands and keep your arms straight, do not bend at the elbow. Do not lean back.

4. Try to keep your arms directly overhead, not forward of your head. Relax your stomach muscles.

5. Hold as directed on your menu.

Fun Facts

This exercise promotes lumbar and thoracic extension through bilateral hip demand.

. . . .

Static Back Knee Pillow Squeezes

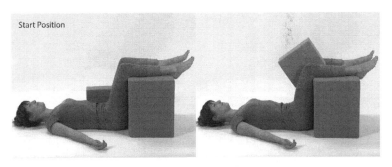

Start Position

Sets = 3, Reps = 20

How to Perform

1. Lie on your back with your legs up over a block or chair.
2. Place a pillow between your knees.
3. Place your arms out to the sides at 45 degrees from your body with palms up.
4. Relax your upper back.
5. Squeeze your knees into the pillow then release.

   Try not to contract your stomach/abdominal muscles while squeezing.
6. Repeat as directed on your menu.

Fun Facts

This exercise stabilizes the pelvis bilaterally. This Static Back position creates horizontal load between shoulder and pelvis, which contributes to thoracic extension by engaging the stabilizers and flexors of the hip. This position helps prevent compensation from occurring while performing other types of muscular work.

Airbench

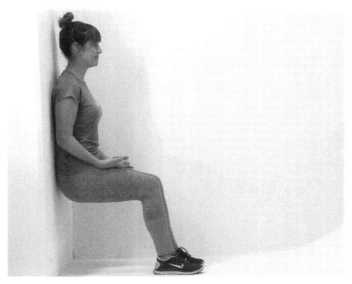

Sets = 1, Reps = 1, Duration = 00:02:00

How to Perform

1. Stand with your back against a wall with feet and knees hip width apart and feet pointed straight.

2. Walk your feet away from the wall while sliding

your body down at the same time. You will be "seated" in an invisible chair, with your knees bent to 105 degrees.

Your hips are just slightly higher than your knees; your ankles are slightly ahead of your knees. Your lower back should be completely flat against the wall.

Your arms can hang down to your sides, or rest your hands gently on your lap.

3. Hold as directed on your menu.

    Keep the weight in your heels, do not press forward on your toes.

4. DO NOT DO THIS E-CISE IN SOCKS!

5. DO THIS EXERCISE IN ATHLETIC SHOES OR ON A YOGA MAT!

Fun Facts

A key component in walking is Quad strength. In this E-cise we are increasing the strength of this muscle group.

SHOPPING LIST

To Have in Pantry at Any Given Time

- Sea Salt
- Herbamare
- Coconut Aminos

- Coconut Milk

- Olive Oil
- Balsamic Vinegar
- Dill
- Granulated Garlic
- Italian Herb Seasoning
- Ground Cumin
- Onion Powder

- White Pepper

- Veggie Pepper
- Blackening Cajun Spice
- Xanthan Gum/ Arrowroot (for baking and thickening soups)
- Dried Basil

- Dried Cherries
- Dried Cranberries
- 14 oz And 32 oz Veggie Broth
- Small Can Hearts Of Palm
- Sliced Almonds
- Pumpkin Seeds
- Pistachios
- Green Lentils
- Small Can Artichoke Hearts
- Red Lentils
- Small Canned Black Bean
- Large & Small Canned Garbanzo
- Brown Basmati Rice
- Quinoa

- Green Split Pea

- Large Can Diced Tomatoes

- Chili Powder
- Crushed Red Pepper
- Lemon Juice
- Green Curry Paste
- Cayenne Pepper

- Tahini
- Sesame Seeds, Unhulled
- Sundried Tomato Bits
- Rice Dream Plain Rice Milk
- Turmeric
- Arrowroot
- Stone-ground Mustard
- Sweet Chili Ginger Sauce

- Small Can White Bean
- Small Can Red Bean

- Pine Nuts
- Small Can Fire Roasted Tomatoes
- Pecans
- Amaranth

- Thyme

- Walnuts

- Sunflower Seeds
- Canned Pumpkin
- Cashews

- Coconut Oil

PERISHABLES

- Kale
- Chard
- Collard
- Carrot
- Celery
- Onion, Red And Yellow
- Garlic
- Spring Mix

- Broccoli
- Zucchini
- Yellow Squash
- Vegan Mayo
- Cucumber
- Frozen Cauliflower
- Raspberries
- Granny Smith Apple
- Pear
- Watercress
- Orange
- Lemon
- Red Cabbage
- Mango
- Frozen Butternut Squash
- Acorn Squash

- Spinach/Arugula Mix
- Ginger Root
- Parsley
- Sweet Potato
- Cremini Mushroom
- Avocado

- Horseradish
- Red/Green Bell Pepper
- Roma Tomato
- Cilantro
- Mint
- Shallot
- Jalapenos
- Strawberries
- Blueberries
- Pink Lady Apple
- Plum
- Fennel
- Lime
- Grapefruit
- Asparagus
- Kiwi
- Butternut Squash

- Crunchy Sprout Mix

- Spaghetti Squash
- Frozen French-cut Green Beans
- Jicama
- Shiitake Mushrooms

WIPING THE SLATE CLEAN

SOUPS

Here's where the rule-breaking begins. I was scared stiff the first time my chef told me to make the soup of the day. What if I didn't cut the mirepoix the proper size? What if I made the wrong roux? My soup would be a total disaster. Then, I found out, all you really need to do in order to make a delightful soup is to just make it. Don't think about anything except the fact that you want a yummy soup. Think about the flavors and textures you want in that soup; toss it in a pot and add some water or stock. Bring it to a boil, reduce to a simmer, and let it cook at least forty-five minutes. You will have a perfect soup every time.

No seriously, food is only as intimidating as you make it up to be, just like anything else in life. You can have fun with it or be scared of it and starve.

Me? I'm always hungry, so I have to cook or else I won't have anything to eat. Have some fun with these soups: they won't bite – promise =)

Black Bean Soup

Vegan ∘ Serves 2 ∘ Gluten Free

1 Large Can Black Beans	1 Small Onion, Finely Diced
3 Garlic Cloves, Finely Diced	1 Pinch Of Crushed Red Pepper
2 Teaspoon Ground Cumin	1 Teaspoon White Pepper
2 Teaspoons Herbamare	1 Tablespoon Olive Oil

1. In A Sauce Pot, Heat Olive Oil On High Heat. When Hot, Add Garlic, Onion And Crushed Red Pepper. Toast Until Onions Are Shiny, Stirring Occasionally. Add Cumin And White Pepper. Toast 2 Minutes.

2. Add Beans With Liquid And 2 Cans Of Water. Add Herbamare And Bring To A Boil.

3. Stir Then Cover And Simmer 10-15 Minutes, Stirring Occasionally.

Red Bean Soup

Vegan ○ Serves 4 ○ Gluten Free

2 Small Cans Red Beans Or Pinto Beans

1 Small Yellow Onion, Diced

3 Garlic Gloves, Finely Diced

1 Pinch Of Crushed Red Pepper

1 Teaspoon Ground Cumin

1 Tablespoon Chili Powder

1 Tablespoon Herbamare

1 Tablespoon Olive Oil

1. In A Soup Pot, Heat Oil On High And Sauté Onion, Garlic And Crushed Red Pepper Until Aromatic. Add Spices And Toast For 1 To 2 Minutes.

2. Pour Undrained Beans Into Pot. Fill Cans With Water And Add To Beans. Bring To A Boil, Reduce To Simmer, Add Herbamare, And Cook 15 To 20 Minutes.

Split Pea Soup

Vegan ∘ Serves 2 ∘ Gluten Free

1 Cup Green Split Peas

1 Small Yellow Onion,
Finely Diced

2 Celery Stalks,
Finely Diced

1 Medium Carrot,
Finely Diced

1 Tablespoon
Herbamare

1. Bring 3 Cups Of Water To A Boil In A Medium Sauce Pot With Veggies. Add Split Peas And Herbamare. Bring Back To A Boil, Then Reduce To Simmer And Cover.

2. Cook 1 Hour Until Peas Are Combined, Stirring Occasionally.

Candida Friendly/Wiping The Slate Clean: Omit Carrots.

Thai Green Curry Soup

Vegan ○ Serves 4 ○ Gluten Free

1 Medium Zucchini, Diced Medium

1 Medium Yellow Squash, Diced Medium

2 Small Carrots, Thinly Sliced

1 Head Of Broccoli, Cut Off Florets

1 Can Coconut Milk

1 Tablespoon Dried Basil

1 Tablespoon Herbamare

1 Teaspoon, Additional To Taste Thai Kitchen Green Curry (Curry Is Spicy, So Taste After First Teaspoon)

½ Cup Red Lentils

½ Cup Quinoa (Avoid In This Stage)

. . . .

1. Prepare All Veggies And Place In Sauce Pot With 4 Cups Of Water. Add Next Four Ingredients And Bring To A Boil.

2. Add Grains And Beans, Then Bring Back To Boil, Reduce To A Simmer, Cover And Cook 40 To 45 Minutes.

Caution: Green Curry Contains Peanut Oil

Creamy Broccoli Soup

Vegan ∘ Serves 2 ∘ Gluten Free

1 Head Of Broccoli, Cut Off Florets

1 Can Coconut Milk

1 Tablespoon Herbamare

1 Teaspoon Xanthan Gum(Optional)

1. In A Sauce Pot, Place Broccoli And Cover With Water. Add Herbamare,

2. Bring To A Boil, Then Cover And Reduce Heat To Simmer. Cook Until Soft, About 20 Minutes.

3. Pour Broth And Broccoli Into A Blender With Xanthan Gum. Blend To Make Smooth And Creamy.

Vegetable Soup

Vegan o Serves 4 o Gluten Free

1 28 Oz. Can Diced Tomatoes

1 Head Broccoli, Cut Off Florets

1 Small Zucchini, Medium Diced

1 Small Yellow Squash, Medium Diced

2 Celery Stalks, Finely Diced

1 Small Yellow Onion, Finely Diced

1 Medium Carrot, Thinly Sliced

1 Tablespoon Herbamare

You May Add:

1 Tablespoon Italian Herbs

1 Tablespoon Granulated Garlic

1 Small Can Beans, Of Choice, Drained

Or At Boiling, Add 1 cup Uncooked Lentils

1. Prepare All Veg And Place In Saucepot.
2. Add Tomatoes (After Step 1) And 6 Cups Of Water. Add Herbamare.
3. Place On Stove, Bring To A Boil, Then Reduce To Simmer. Cook 45 To 50 Minutes. Serve.

Pumpkin White Bean Soup

Vegan ○ Serves 2 ○ Gluten Free

1- 15 Oz. Can Pumpkin

1- 15 Oz. Can White Beans

1- 15 Oz. Can Coconut Milk

1 Tablespoon Walnuts

1 Tablespoon Unsweetened Shredded Coconut (Optional)

Herbamare To Taste

1. Place Pumpkin, Undrained White Beans, Nuts, Coconut And Half The Can Of Coconut Milk In A Blender.
2. Begin To Mix On Medium To Blend And Go Higher If Needed.
3. Add More Coconut Milk To Thin Out, If Desired.
4. Season To Taste With Herbamare. Warm Over Medium Heat. Be Careful Not To Scorch.

Chia Limeade

Makes 8 Cups

1 Tablespoon Chia
Seeds

2 Limes, Juiced

7 Cups Water

6 Packets 100% Stevia

1. Soak The Chia Seeds For 10 Minutes In The Water.
2. Add Lime Juice And Stevia. Stir To Mix And Enjoy.

Wiping The Slate Clean

. . . .

Cold Dishes

I didn't want to call these dishes "salads," because that term to me implies they are already done and ready to eat. These dishes may be used as a starter, an accompaniment to a meal, on top of a bed of salad greens, as salsas, toppings for chips, their possibilities are endless.

Where there is room, I have offered suggestions to make these recipes your own with variations, and/or food pairings to make your life simpler. I've attempted to give you some food combinations for complete proteins. Also, especially when it comes to raw dishes, I attempt to properly combine foods as much as possible.

Avocado Salsa

Vegan ∘ Serves 6 ∘ Gluten Free

3 Ripe Avocados, Pit Removed And Diced

1 Medium Tomato, Small Dice

3 Garlic Cloves, Minced

½ Tsp Sea Salt +

2 Tablespoons Lemon Juice

½ Bunch Cilantro, Chopped (Optional)

1 Pinch Of Crushed Red Pepper

1. Chop Garlic And ½ Teaspoon Sea Salt. Add Crushed Red Pepper.

2. Prepare Avocado And Tomato, Place In Bowl. Put Garlic On Top Of Avocado And Cilantro. Pour Lemon Juice Over Veg. Stir To Combine.

3. Season With Sea Salt To Taste.

Cilantro Ginger Green Beans

Vegan ○ Serves 2 ○ Gluten Free

1 Pound Fresh Green Beans

1 Bunch Cilantro

3 Garlic Cloves, Peeled

2" Piece Of Ginger

1/2 Cup Apple Cider Vinegar

1/2 Cup Coconut Aminos

1/3 Cup Olive Oil

1. Clean Green Beans. Bring A Large Pot Of Water To A Boil. Add Green Beans. Bring Back To A Boil And Cook 5 To 7 Minutes. Drain And Rinse With Cold Water To Cool.

2. While Beans Are Cooling, Add To Blender: Garlic, Cilantro, Ginger, Vinegar, Aminos, And Olive Oil. Blend To Smooth.

3. Toss Half Of Dressing With Green Beans. Save The Other Half Of Dressing For More Beans Or Use As A Fish/Chicken Marinade Or Salad Dressing.

Hummus

Vegan ○ Serves 6 ○ Gluten Free

1 Large Can Garbanzo Beans

3 Garlic Cloves, Peeled

1 Tablespoon Lemon Juice

1 Teaspoon Sea Salt

1/8 Tsp Cayenne Pepper

½ Cup Tahini

1. Place All Ingredients Into A Food Processor Or A Medium Bowl.

2. Turn On High To Blend. If Needed, Pulse To Combine First. If More Liquid Is Needed, Add Water, 2 Tablespoons At A Time To Make Smoother. If Using A Bowl, You'll Be Using A Hand Blender.

3. Serve With Raw Veggies.

White Bean Salad

Vegan ∘ Serves 2 ∘ Gluten Free

1 Can Northern Beans, Drained

1 Small Carrot, Finely Diced

1 Celery Stalk, Finely Diced

1 Small Tomato, Diced

½ Small Red Onion, Finely Diced

1/3 Cup Lemon Juice

¼ Cup Olive Oil

½ Teaspoon Herbamare

½ Teaspoon Sea Salt

1 Teaspoon Granulated Garlic

1. Rinse And Drain Beans, Place In Medium Bowl. Prepare All Veggies And Add To Beans.

2. Combine Next Five Ingredients In A Separate Bowl And Whisk Together.

3. Pour Over Bean/Veggie Mixture And Toss To Combine.

4. Let Set At Room Temperature For 20 Minutes To Marinate Before Serving.

5. May Add A Small Bunch Of Chopped Parsley Or Watercress.

Candida Friendly: Leave Out Tomato And Carrot

Mock Ranch Dip

Vegan ○ Serves 4 ○ Gluten Free

1 Cup Soaked Raw Cashews

1/2 Cup Water

2 Teaspoons Freshly Squeezed Lemon Juice

1/2 Teaspoon Garlic Powder

1/2 Teaspoon Onion Powder

1/4 Tsp Salt

2 Tablespoons Minced Fresh Chives Or Green Onion

1 Tablespoon Minced Fresh Basil, Or 1 Teaspoon Dried

1 Tablespoon Minced Fresh Dill, Or 1 Teaspoon Dried Dill Weed

1. 1. Put The Cashews, Water, Lemon Juice, Garlic Powder, Onion Powder, And Salt Into A Blender And Process Until Smooth.

2. 2. Stop Occasionally To Scrape Down The Blender Jar With A Rubber Spatula.

3. 3. Add The Chives, Basil, And Dill, Then Pulse Briefly To Mix.

4. 4. Chill For At Least 30 Minutes Before Serving. Store In A Sealed Container In The Refrigerator. Will Keep For 5 Days.

Cauliflower Tabouli

Vegan ○ Serves 2 ○ Gluten Free

½ Head Cauliflower, Chopped Fine

1 Bag Baby Spinach, Chopped

1 Small Red Onion, Finely Diced (Or Shallot)

1 Roma Tomato, Small Dice

½ Cup Pine Nuts

1 Lemon, Juiced

1 Teaspoon Each Of: Sea Salt, Granulated Garlic

1/3 Cup Olive Oil

1. Chop Cauliflower In Half, And Chop Into Tiny Pieces. Place Into A Medium Bowl.

2. Chop Spinach And Add To Cauliflower, Followed By Onion And Tomato.

3. Add Pine Nuts, Salt And Garlic.

4. Drizzle With Lemon Juice And Olive Oil. Mix To Combine. Enjoy.

Cucumber & Watercress Salad

Candida Friendly ∘ Serves 2 ∘ Gluten Free

1 Bunch Watercress	1 Lime, Juiced
1 Seedless Cucumber	¼ Cup Olive Oil
½ Small Red Onion	½ Teaspoon Herbamare
½ Red Bell Pepper	

1. Wash Watercress And Remove Thick Stems. Transfer To A Bowl.
2. Halve Cucumber And Thinly Slice Into Half Moons. Add To Watercress.
3. Thinly Slice Red Onion And Small Diced Red Pepper. Add To Watercress/ Cucumber Mixture.
4. Whisk Together Lime Juice, Olive Oil And Herbamare. Drizzle Over Salad And Toss.

Party Slaw

Vegan ∘ Serves 2 ∘ Gluten Free

¼ Head Cabbage, Shredded

1 Small Yellow Squash, Grated

½ Small Sweet Potato, Peeled And Grated

1 Avocado, Diced

1 Lemon, Juiced

1 - 2 Teaspoons Herbamare

1/3 Cup Pistachios, Chopped

½ Teaspoon White Pepper

1. Prep All Veg And Place In A Large Bowl.

2. Add Lemon Juice, Herbamare, And White Pepper. Toss To Mix And Serve.

Broccoli, Avocado, Pistachio

Vegan ○ Serves 2 ○ Gluten Free

1 Broccoli Crown,
   Separated Into Florets

1 Avocado, Diced

½ Cup Pistachios,
   Shelled And Chopped

1 Roma Tomato, Diced

1 Lemon, Juiced

¼ Cup Red Onion, Diced

1. Prep All Veg And Place Into A Medium Bowl.

2. Pour Lemon Juice Over Mixture. Toss Together And Enjoy.

Artichoke Garbanzo

Vegan ∘ Serves 2 ∘ Gluten Free

1 - 14 Oz. Can Artichoke Hearts, Quartered And Drained

1 - 15.5 Oz. Can Garbanzo Beans, Drained

¼ Cup Red Onion, Small Dice

½ Small Bunch Parsley, Chopped

1 Teaspoon Sea Salt

½ Teaspoon Black Pepper

¼ Cup Raw Apple Cider Vinegar

2 Tablespoons Olive Oil

1. Drain Beans And Artichoke Hearts And Place Together In A Medium Bowl.
2. Prep Onion And Parsley And Add To The Bean Mixture.
3. Sprinkle Salt, Pepper, Vinegar, And Olive Oil Over Ingredients.
4. Toss To Mix, Let Mixture Set 20 Minutes And Serve.

Options: *Add 2 - 4 Oz. Goat Cheese (No Longer Vegan – Pygmalion), 2 Small Roma Tomatoes, Diced (Vocabulary), ½ Red Bell Pepper, Diced, 2 Chopped Green Onions, Including The White Part. And/Or Fresh Thyme , Oregano Or Basil.*

Kale Chop

Vegan ○ Serves 4 ○ Gluten Free

1 Head Kale, Small Chop

1 Zucchini, Shredded

1 Small Red Onion, Small Dice

1 Carrot, Small Dice

1 Red Bell Pepper, Small Dice

1 Yellow Squash, Shredded

1 Can Garbanzo Beans, Drained

1 Lemon, Juiced

1 Teaspoon Sea Salt

1 Teaspoon Black Pepper

1 Tablespoon Olive Oil

1. Wash And Prep All Veg. Place In A Large Bowl.

2. Juice The Lemon And Drizzle Over Veg. Sprinkle With Salt And Pepper. Finish With A Drizzle Of Olive Oil.

3. Massage Lemon Juice And Seasonings Into Kale, Mix For About 3 Minutes. Enjoy!

Yellow Squash And Crunchy Sprouts

Vegan ∘ Serves 2 ∘ Gluten Free

2 Yellow Squash, Small Dice

1 Container Crunchy Sprout Mix

1 Bunch Lacinato Kale, Chopped

1 Red Pepper, Thinly Sliced

1 Lemon, Juiced

2 Teaspoons Herbamare

. . . .

1. Place Chopped Kale Into A Medium Mixing Bowl.

2. Dice Yellow Squash To A Small Size And Add To Kale. Add Sliced Red Pepper.

3. Sprinkle Crunchy Sprouts On Top, Followed By Herbamare And Lemon Juice.

4. Toss To Mix. Enjoy.

Zucchini, Avocado With Cilantro

Vegan ○ Serve 2 ○ Gluten Free

2 Zucchini, Shredded

2 Avocados, Diced

1 Garlic Cloves, Minced

1 Small Bunch Cilantro, Chopped

1 Lime, Juiced

½ Cup Pumpkin Seeds

Sea Salt, To Taste

1 Pinch Of Crushed Red Pepper

1 Small Jalapeno, Minced (Optional)

Prep All Veg And Place Into A Bowl. Pour Lime Juice Over And Gently Toss To Mix. Season To Taste With Sea Salt.

Vinaigrette

1 Cup Braggs Apple
Cider Vinegar

1cup Water

1 Tablespoon.
Herbamare

1 Teaspoon Onion Salt

1 Teaspoon Celery Salt

25 Drops Liquid Stevia

Pour All Ingredients Into An 18-Ounce Jar Or Cruet.
Shake Well And Refrigerate Until Ready To Use.

Asian Dressing

1 Cup Braggs Apple Cider Vinegar

1 Cup Water

1 Teaspoon Garlic Salt

1 Teaspoon Onion Salt

1 Teaspoon Chinese Five Spice

¼ Cup Freshly Squeezed Lemon Juice

25 Drops Liquid Stevia

Pour All Ingredients Into An 18-Ounce Jar Or Cruet. Shake Well And Store In Refrigerator Until Use.

Wiping The Slate Clean

Hot Dishes

An important note needs to be made here. Under hot dishes, you will see only three that are veggies and then there are a large number of meat and fish dishes. Any of the meat and fish dishes can have the animal product replaced with beans, seeds, and/or nuts for plant-based protein. You will notice substitutions at the end of each recipe. Animal product is not a necessary ingredient to have balanced eating and I like to provide options for those who are looking for a more plant-based lifestyle without using soy, wheat gluten, or manufactured protein products.

Oven Roasted Veggies

Vegan ∘ Serves 2-4 ∘ Gluten Free

1 Tablespoon Each Italian Herbs, Granulated Garlic

1 Tsp Sea Salt

1 Head Broccoli, Cut Into Florets

1 Medium Zucchini, Cut Into Bite-Sized Pieces

1 Medium Yellow Squash, Cut Into Bite-Sized Pieces

1 Large Carrot, Cut Into ½" Slices

1 8 Oz. Package Mushrooms, Quartered

Coconut Or Olive Oil

1. Preheat Oven To 425 Degrees.

2. Place All Prepped Veggies Into A 9"X 13" Baking Pan.

3. Sprinkle Seasonings Over Veggies. Drizzle Oil Over Veggies To Lightly Coat. Toss To Mix.

4. Bake At 425 Degrees For 20-25 Minutes, Stirring Twice.

Note: *Sizes Of Veggies Will Vary For Cooking Time, I.E. To Evenly Cook Everything, Carrots Need To Be Cut Thinner Than Squash Due To Density.*

Wilted Greens

Vegan ○ Serves 2 ○ Gluten Free

1 Bunch Kale, Collards, Or Swiss Chard, Chopped Bite-Sized

1 Small Yellow Onion, Small Dice

3 Garlic Cloves, Minced

1 Pinch Crushed Red Pepper

1 Tablespoon Olive Oil

Coconut Aminos

1. Prepare All Veg And Keep Separate.

2. In A Large Sauté Pan, Heat Oil On High Heat. When You Can Feel The Heat Of The Pan, Add Garlic And Crushed Red Pepper. Toast Until You Can Smell The Garlic.

3. Add Onions And Sauté Until Shiny.

4. Add Greens And 2 Tablespoons Of Water. Cover.

5. Cook Until Greens Are Wilted, Stirring Occasionally. Do Not Overcook. Greens Should Be Deep Green In Color, Not Olive Green.

6. Remove From Heat And Season To Taste With Coconut Aminos. Serve

Snow Pea W/Ginger And Bok Choy

Vegan ○ Serves 2 ○ Gluten Free

½ Pound Snow Peas, Cut On The Diagonal

4 Baby Bok Choy, Cut In ¼-Inch Pieces

½-Inch Piece Ginger, Minced

Veggie Stock (Optional)

3 Garlic Cloves, Minced

Olive Oil Or Sesame Oil

Sea Salt

Crushed Red Pepper

Coconut Aminos

1. Prep All Veg. Peel Garlic And Ginger. Mince On Top Of ½ Teaspoon Sea Salt And A Dash Of Crushed Red Pepper.

2. Heat 1 Tablespoon Oil In A Large Sauté Pan. Add Garlic/Ginger Mix, Toast 30 Seconds, Until Aromatic.

3. Add Snow Peas And Bok Choy With 2 Tablespoons Of Broth Or Water. Cover And Steam 3-5 Minutes.

4. Remove Cover And Stir. Veggies Should Be Cooked, But Firm.

5. Season With Aminos Or Salt And Pepper.

Wiping The Slate Clean

Meat And Seafood

Zucchini, Cilantro, Chicken And Ginger

Serves 1 ∘ Gluten Free

1 Large Zucchini

3 Oz. Chicken, Thinly Sliced

¾ Bunch Cilantro, Chopped

1 Teaspoon Garlic Salt

1-Inch Piece Of Ginger, Minced

3 Tablespoons Asian Vinaigrette

1. Marinade Chicken With 1 Tablespoon Vinaigrette In A Ziploc Baggie While Preparing Veggies.

2. Slice Zucchini Into 1-Inch Half Moons. Chop Cilantro And Mince Ginger.

3. Heat Sauté Pan On Medium High.

4. Add All Ingredients To Pan With Remaining Vinaigrette. To Steam, Cover With Lid. Cook 5-7 Minutes, Stirring Occasionally. Add More Vinaigrette Or Water To Assist With Cooking, If Needed.

Options- *Use 3 – 4 Baby Bok Choy, Cut In Quarters, Along With 1/2 Cup Of Cashews Or Almonds, In Place Of Chicken.*

Rosemary Fish And Asparagus

Serves One ○ Gluten Free

3 Oz. Fish Of Choice

1 Teaspoon Lemon Juice

2 Cups Asparagus/1 Bu, Trimmed

1 Teaspoon Granulated Garlic

1 Teaspoon Rosemary

½ Teaspoon Sea Salt

1 Teaspoon Herbamare

Cider Vinegar

- -

1. Heat A George Foreman Grill To Medium High. Season Fish With Rosemary, Sea Salt And Granulated Garlic.

2. Toss Asparagus With Herbamare And Cider Vinegar.

3. When Hot, Place Asparagus On Grill First. Cook For 3 Minutes, Then Add Fish.

4. Cook 5-7 Minutes Until Done.

5. Alternately, Preheat Oven To 425 Degrees. Place Seasoned Asparagus On Top Of Fish On A Rectangular Piece Of Parchment Paper Or Foil. Wrap Fish And Veg Into A Package And Bake 15-18 Minutes.

Ginger Chicken W/Snow Peas And Shiitake

Serves 2 ∘ Gluten Free

½ Pound Of Chicken Tenders Or Breasts

3 Cups Snow Peas

6 Shiitake Mushrooms

1-Inch Piece Ginger, Minced

½ Tablespoon Sesame Oil

½ Tsp Sea Salt

½ Tablespoon Olive Oil

1 Tablespoon Asian Seasoning

1. Place Sauté Pan On Medium High Heat.

2. While Pan Is Heating, Mince The Ginger On Top Of ½ Teaspoon Sea Salt.

3. When You Can Feel The Heat In The Pan By Placing Your Hand Over The Center Of It (*Over* Not In), Add Oils, Then Chicken, Ginger, Snow Peas, And Mushrooms. Stir.

4. Depending On The Pan, You May Need To Add 2 Tablespoons Of Water, So As Not To Burn Anything.

5. Cover And Stir Occasionally, Until Chicken Is Cooked, About 7 - 9 Minutes. Season With Asian Seasoning And Enjoy.

Options – *In Place Of Chicken, Use 1 Bunch Of Kale Chopped, And A Can Of Drained Black Beans.*

Shrimp, Squash And Sausage

Serves 2 ○ Gluten Free

4 To 5 Yellow Crookneck Squash (Or Zucchini), Sliced

1 Onion, Finely Chopped

½ Pound Italian Sausage

2/3 Pound Raw Shrimp (Peeled/Deveined/Tails Off)

Sea Salt, Pepper, Cajun Seasoning

1 Teaspoon Olive Oil

1. Heat Olive Oil In Sauté Pan Over Medium-High Heat.

2. Remove Sausage From Casing And Sauté With Onion, Until Onion Is Shiny.

3. Add Squash And Sauté Until Caramelized.

4. Season With Cajun Spice And Add Shrimp. Cook Until Shrimp Are Opaque.

Beef, Snap Pea, And Shiitake Stir Fry

Serves 2 ○ Gluten Free

1/2 Pound Stir-Fry Beef

3 Cups Sugar Snap Peas

8 Shiitake Mushrooms, Thinly Sliced

½-Inch Piece Of Ginger

1 Garlic Clove

Sea Salt

Asian Spice/5 Spice (Optional)

Olive And/Or Sesame Oil

1. Remove Woody Stems From Shiitakes And Slice Caps Thin.
2. Peel And Mince Garlic And Ginger Together Over ½ Teaspoon Sea Salt And Crushed Red Pepper (Optional).
3. Heat Sauté Pan Over Medium-High Heat.
4. Add Oil, Ginger/Garlic Mixture, Meat, And Veggies.
5. Stir Fry 4 To 6 Minutes, Until Meat Is Cooked. Add Asian Seasoning Or Tamari To Taste.

Options – *Instead Of Beef, Try Adding 1 Large Portobello Mushroom, Sliced, And A Medium Zucchini Sliced Into ¼ Inch Half-Moons. I Also Like To Add ½ Bunch Of Chopped Kale Or Baby Spinach When I Don't Want To Work Too Hard, Along With Sunflower Seeds.*

Chicken With Sesame Broccoli

Serves 2 ∘ Gluten Free

½ Pound Chicken Tenders

1 Full Head Broccoli, Cut Off Florets

1 Tablespoon Sesame Oil

1 Tablespoon Sesame Ginger Blend

Sesame Seeds

¼ Cup Chicken Stock

Coconut Aminos To Taste

1. Heat Oil On Medium High Heat. Add Broccoli And Chicken.

2. Saute, Add Chicken Stock And Cover To Cook 5 Minutes.

3. Add Sesame Seeds, Cook 2 More Minutes. Season To Taste With Coconut Aminos.

Options - *Again, Here I Would Add 6 Baby Bella Mushrooms, Cut In Quarters, And A Dark Leafy Green Such As Kale Or Swill Chard, Chopped, 1 Bunch.*

Ginger Lime Chicken

Serves 2 ∘ Gluten Free

1/2 Pound Chicken Tenders

1 Medium Zucchini, Sliced Into Half Moons

1 Red Bell Pepper, Sliced Thin

1-Inch Piece Ginger, Minced

1 Clove Garlic, Minced

1 Lime, Juiced

Coconut Amino's To Taste

1 Tbsp Olive Oil

1. Prep Veg.
2. Peel And Mince Garlic And Ginger Together Over ½ Tsp Sea Salt.
3. Heat Olive Oil Over Medium High Heat. Add Chicken, Ginger/Garlic Mix And Zucchini.
4. Cover, Stir Fry 5 Minutes, Stirring Occasionally. When Chicken Is Almost Done, Add Peppers And Lime Juice. Cook 2 More Minutes.
5. Season To Taste With Aminos.

Mediterranean Roasted Fish

Serves 2 ∘ Gluten Free

8 Oz. Grouper Or Other Meaty White Fish

1 Small Jar Artichoke Hearts, Drained

1sm Bag Baby Spinach

1 Bag Frozen Broccoli Florets

1 Teaspoon Granulated Garlic

1 Teaspoon Herbamare

1-2 Tablespoons Olive Oil

1. Preheat Over 425 Degrees.
2. In Cake Pan Or Large Cookie Sheet, Place All Ingredients, Sprinkling The Seasonings On Top, Finishing With The Olive Oil.
3. Toss Gently To Mix. Bake In Oven 20 To 25 Minutes.

Options – *Toss In Some White Beans, Cannellini, Or Northern In Place Of The Fish.*

Spring Rolls

Serves 1 ∘ Gluten Free

3 ½ Oz. Chicken, Shrimp, Or Crab

1 Small Cucumber/1/4 Regular Cucumber, Seeded And Sliced In Quarters

4 Spears Asparagus, Steamed (Or Cooked With Other Asparagus)

1 Head Boston Lettuce

1 Cup Chopped Romaine Or Rest Of Boston Lettuce

Asian Dressing Used As Dipping Sauce

Chinese Five Spice

Herbamare

1. Use Four Large Outer Leaves For Wrappers. Chop Remaining Lettuce. Set Aside.

2. Steam Protein And Asparagus, With Asparagus On Top Layer. Cook 6 To 10 Minutes; Place In Fridge To Cool.

3. Chop Chicken/Shellfish; Mix With Chopped Lettuce And Season With Five-Spice And Herbamare.

4. Take 1 Asparagus, 1 Cucumber, And ¼ Lettuce Mix, Place In Lettuce Cup. Roll 'Burrito' Style And Dip In Vinaigrette.

Options – *Add Crunchy Sprout Mix For The Meat, And Shred A Carrot, Yum!*

Chinese Chicken With Sesame Broccoli

Serves 2 ○ Gluten Free

½ Pound Chicken Tenders

1 Full Head Broccoli, Cut Off Florets

1 Tablespoon Sesame Oil

1 Tsp Asian Seasoning/ Five Spice

¼ Cup Chicken Stock

Coconut Aminos To Taste

1. Heat Oil On Medium High Heat. Add Broccoli And Chicken.
2. Saute, Add Chicken Stock, And Cover To Cook 5 Minutes.
3. Add Sesame Seeds, Cook 2 More Minutes. Season To Taste With Coconut Aminos.

Options – 1 To 2 Large Portobello Mushrooms Slices, Along With 2 Tablespoons Sliced Almonds For Texture. And, Of Course, Substitute Veggie Broth.

The Vocabulary

Ahhhhh, freedom! You have made it! It wasn't so bad? Look how clear your skin is and feel how much more energy you have! So now we are adding fruits and animal protein back in. I am providing you with more (yes more) veggie and fruit recipes because it is so easy to make a protein and you need six to twelve veggie servings a day. Hey, it's your health and it's your life. I'm here as your food companion. Take the protein recipes from detox section and add these recipes with it. Do you have to add animal product? No. I believe it is everyone's option to know how their body communicates with the food they are eating. Isn't that the point of this book?

Following three weeks in The **Vocabulary**, in *Pygmalion*, you will notice there are some grain-related recipes. You will be using these if that is what you and your practitioner have agreed upon. It is an honor system that you are on in this program. It's your choice what you do with your health. Me, I'm here to make sure it is tasty. I am also here to set you up for optimal success.

Vocabulary

Soups

Creamy Tomato Basil Soup

Vegan ∘ Serves 4 ∘ Gluten Free

1 - 28 Oz. Can Diced Tomatoes

1 Tablespoon Dried Basil

1 Tablespoon Herbamare

1 Teaspoon Xanthan Gum (Optional)

1 Can Coconut Milk

1. In 4 Quart Sauce Pot, Put The First Three Ingredients, Plus Half A Can Of Water.

2. Bring To A Boil Over High Heat, Reduce To Simmer, Then Cover And Cook 20 Minutes.

3. Puree In Blender Or With A Hand Blender With Xanthan Gum.

Roasted Tomato And Cauliflower Soup

Vegan ∘ Serves 2 ∘ Gluten Free

1 – 15 Oz. Can Fire Roasted Tomatoes

1 – 15 Oz. Can Veggie Stock/Broth

1 – 9oz Bag Frozen Cauliflower

1 Teaspoon Herbamare

1. In A Medium Soup Pot, Place Tomatoes And Broth. Bring To A Boil

2. When Boiling, Add Cauliflower And Herbamare.

3. Cook 15 To 20 Minutes Until Cauliflower Is At Desired Tenderness.

4. Season To Taste And Enjoy

5. Make It Yours By Blending Half Of The Soup To Make It Thicker Or By Adding Coconut Milk.

Spicy Mango Ginger Soup

Serves 2 ∘ Gluten Free

1 Large Mango, Peeled And Diced

1 Chili Pepper, Seeded

1/2 Cup Chopped Sweet Yellow Onion

1/2 Cup Water

Juice Of 1 Lime

1/2 Tsp Grated Fresh Ginger

1. Peel And Dice Mango.
2. Place All Ingredients In Blender.
3. Blend Until Smooth And Creamy.

Gazpacho

Vegan ∘ Serves 2 ∘ Gluten Free

3 Medium Tomatoes

1 Small Cucumber

½ Small Red Onion

¼ Cup Cilantro

½ Red Bell Pepper

1 Garlic Clove

1 Lime Juiced

1 Teaspoon Chili Powder

1 Jalapeño, Seeded

Sea Salt To Taste

1. Small Diced Tomatoes. Put In Mixing Bowl.

2. Seed And Dice Cucumber And Bell Pepper. Finely Dice Red Onion. Chop Cilantro. Place In A Mixing Bowl. Seed And Dice Jalapeño. Add To Bowl.

3. Combine Rest Of Ingredients, Pour Into Blender 2 Cups At A Time And Blend At High Speed For 20 – 30 Seconds.

White Gazpacho

Vegan ∘ Serves 2 ∘ Gluten Free

1 Tablespoon Olive Oil

1 Cup Leeks, White And Light-Green Parts Only, Thinly Sliced Crosswise

2 English Cucumbers - Peeled, Quartered, And Chopped

8 Green Grapes

1/4 Cup Slivered Blanched Almonds

1 Lime Juiced

1- 1/2 Cup Cold Water, Or More As Needed

Sea Salt, To Taste

1 Pinch Cayenne Pepper, Or To Taste

1. Heat 1 Tablespoon Olive Oil In A Saucepan Over Medium-Low Heat. Cook And Stir Leeks Until Soft, 10 To 15 Minutes. Remove To A Plate And Allow To Cool.

2. Place Cucumbers In A Blender With Grapes, Almonds, 1 Tablespoon Olive Oil, Salt, Lime Juice, Cooled Leeks, And Water. Puree Until Smooth, About 1 Minute. Strain Through A Fine Mesh Sieve. Cover And Chill For 1 To 2 Hours.

3. Taste And Season With Salt And Cayenne Pepper. If Needed, Add Some More Lime Juice.

Mango Gazpacho

Vegan ○ Serves 4 ○ Gluten Free

2 Cups 1/4-Inch-Diced Fresh Mangoes

2 Cups Orange Juice

1 Seedless Cucumber, Diced Into 1/4-Inch Pieces

1 Small Red Bell Pepper, Seeded And Diced Into 1/4-Inch Pieces

1 Small Onion, Diced Into 1/4-Inch Pieces

2 Medium Garlic Cloves, Minced

1 Small Jalapeno Pepper, Seeded And Minced (Optional)

3 Tablespoons Fresh Lime Juice

2 Tablespoons Chopped Fresh Parsley, Basil Or Cilantro, Salt And Freshly Ground Black Pepper

1. Process Mangoes, Orange Juice And Oil In A Blender Or Food Processor Until Pureed. Transfer To A Medium Bowl, Along With Remaining Ingredients. Season With Salt And Pepper To Taste. Refrigerate Until Ready To Serve. (Can Be Made Several Hours Before Serving.)

Peach Gazpacho

Vegan ○ Serves 4 ○ Gluten Free

1/2 To 3/4 Cups Water

6 Ripe Peaches (About 2 - 1/2 Pounds), Peeled, Halved, Pitted, And Cut Into Chunks

1/2 Medium Cucumber, Peeled, Seeded, And Cut Into Chunks

1 Small Garlic Clove, Minced

1 Tablespoon Champagne Vinegar, Plus More To Taste

Sea Salt & Freshly Ground Pepper

2 Tablespoons Coarsely Chopped Fresh Flat-Leaf Parsley Or Cilantro

1. Pulse 1/2 Cup Water, The Peaches, Cucumber, Garlic, Vinegar, Oil, 1/2 Teaspoon Salt, And 1/4 Teaspoon Pepper In A Food Processor Until Coarsely Pureed. Thin With More Water If Desired. Refrigerate For At Least 2 Hours.

Vocabulary Cold Dishes

Plum, Pepper And Cilantro

Vegan ∘ Serves 4 ∘ Gluten Free

1-½ To 2 Pounds Plums, Diced

1 Bunch Cilantro, Chopped

1 Small Green Pepper, Diced Small

1 Small Red Bell Pepper, Diced Small

1 Small Red Onion, Finely Diced

½ Teaspoon Crushed Red Pepper, Optional

2 Limes, Juiced

1. Dice Plums, Peppers And Onions. Place In A Medium Bowl.
2. Rough Chop Cilantro And Add To Fruit Mixture.
3. Sprinkle Crushed Red Pepper And Lime Juice Over Fruit. Toss To Combine. Chill 20 Minutes And Serve.

Zucchini Salad

Vegan ○ Serves 2-4 ○ Gluten Free

¾ - 1 Pound Zucchini, Medium Dice

½ Pound Yellow Squash, Medium Dice

4 Roma Tomato, Medium Dice

1 Medium Green Bell Pepper, Medium Dice

1 Teaspoon Sea Salt

3 Garlic Cloves, Minced

1/4 Teaspoon Crushed Red Pepper

1/3 Cup White Or Red Wine Vinegar

1/3 Cup Olive Oil

1 Tablespoon Frontier Italian Herb Seasonings

1. Prep All Veggies And Place In A Medium Salad Bowl.

2. Mince Garlic With A Pinch Of Salt And Crushed Red Pepper. Sprinkle Over Veg.

3. Mix Herbs, Vinegar And Olive Oil In A Small Bowl And Pour Over Veg. Toss Together And Serve.

Watercress Salad

Vegan ∘ Serves 2 ∘ Gluten Free

2 Bunches Watercress,
Roughly Chopped

1 Medium Cucumber,
Seeded, Small Dice

1 Medium Carrot, Small
Dice

1 Small Red Onion,
Finely Diced

1/4 Cup Lemon Juice

2 Tablespoons Olive Oil

2 Teaspoons
Herbamare

1. Prepare All Veg And Place In A Bowl.

2. Whisk Together Lemon Juice, Olive Oil And
   Herbamare. Pour Over Watercress.

3. Lightly Toss To Combine And Serve.

Lentil Salad

Vegan ∘ Serves 4 ∘ Gluten Free

1 Cup Lentils

1 Small Red Onion, Finely Diced

1 Small Carrot, Finely Diced

1 Celery Stalk, Finely Diced

1/4 Cup Sun-Dried Tomatoes

Dressing

1/3 Cup Coconut Aminos

1/3 Cup Balsamic Vinegar

1 1/4 Cup Olive Oil

2 Teaspoons Italian Herbs

1. In A Medium Sauce Pot, Bring 3 Cups Of Water To A Boil. Add Lentils. Bring Back To A Boil, Reduce To Simmer And Cook 20 Minutes, Until Lentils Are Tender To Bite. Drain And Rinse Lentils With Cool Water Until Water Runs Clear. Let Cool To Room Temperature.

2. While Lentils Are Cooking, Prepare Veg.

3. Combine Dressing Ingredients In A Separate Bowl And Whisk Together.

4. When Lentils Are Cool, Add To Veg And Pour Dressing Over. Stir To Combine.

5. Let Salad Set For 20 Minutes And Serve.

Given To Me By Pam Brown.

Ginger, Pear And Watercress

Vegan ○ Serves 4 ○ Gluten Free

1 ½ -2 Pounds Pears, Slice

Or 1 Pound Pear And 3 Kiwi, Peeled And Diced

2" Piece Of Ginger, Peeled

1 Bunch Watercress, Chopped

1 Orange, Juiced Or 2 Limes, Juiced

1. Dice Pears And/Or Kiwi In A Medium Bowl.
2. Rough Chop Watercress And Add To Fruit.
3. With A Hand Grater, Grate Ginger Over Fruit/ Green Mix.
4. Pour Juiced Fruit Over And Toss To Combine. Chill 20 Minutes And Serve.

This Is Great As A Starter Or Palate Cleanser. Yummy At Breakfast Time, Too, Or Over Grilled Fish.

Apple Fennel W/Lemon

Vegan ○ Serves 2 ○ Gluten Free

2 Fuji Apples, Small Dice

1 Bulb Fennel, Julienned

1 Red Bell Pepper, Minced

1 Lemon, Juiced And Zested

1 Teaspoon Herbamare

1. Prep All Veg And Place In A Medium Bowl.
2. Zest Lemon And Then Juice It.
3. Chop Some Of The Fennel 'Pollen' And Add To Mix.
4. Season With Herbamare And Lemon Juice. Toss To Combine And Enjoy.

Apple Kale

Vegan ∘ Serves 2 ∘ Gluten Free

1 Bunch Kale, Chopped

2 Fuji Apples, Small Dice

1 Lemon, Juiced

1 Carrot, Shredded

2 Tablespoons Chopped Walnuts

1 Teaspoon Herbamare

1. Clean All Produce And Bring To Room Temperature.

2. Dice Apples And Place In A Bowl With 1 Cup Water And 1 Teaspoon Lemon Juice To Prevent Yellowing.

3. Chop Kale And Set In A Medium Bowl. Drain Apples And Add To Kale. Shred Carrot On A Grater And Add To Bowl.

4. Sprinkle Walnuts And Herbamare Over Ingredients.

5. Drizzle Lemon Juice Over Veggies And Fruit And Gently Massage Ingredients Together For 2 – 3 Minutes.

Rainbow Rave

Vegan ○ Serves 2 ○ Gluten Free

1sm Bag Baby Spinach

1 Blood Orange, Segmented

1 Red Pear, Small Dice

2 Zucchini, Shredded

1 Small Shallot, Minced

1 Teaspoon Sea Salt

2 Teaspoons Olive Oil

Fresh Ground Black Pepper

1 Teaspoon Fresh Mint, Cut Chiffonade

1. Place Baby Spinach In A Medium Bowl.
2. Place The Box Grater Over The Spinach And Shred Zucchini.
3. Dice Pear And Add.
4. Mince Shallot And Add To Ingredients.
5. Peel The Blood Orange With A Paring Knife And Cut Into Segments, Adding Them To The Spinach Combination.
6. Season With Sea Salt, Pepper And Mint. Drizzle With Olive Oil And Remaining Juice From The Orange.
7. Toss And Enjoy.

Peach Delight

Vegan ∘ Serves 2 ∘ Gluten Free

2 Peaches, Sliced

1 Tablespoon Mint, Chiffonade

1 Lemon, Juiced

1 Tablespoon Ginger, Minced

1 Cucumber, Seeded And Diced

1 Shallot, Thinly Sliced

2 Teaspoons Herbamare

1. Slice The Cucumber Down The Middle Lengthwise And Remove Seeds With A Teaspoon. Dice And Place In Medium Bowl.
2. Cut Peach In Half And Cut Into 6 -8 Slices.
3. Prep Shallot, Mint And Ginger.
4. Sprinkle With Herbamare And Drizzle With Lemon Juice.
5. Toss Lightly And Enjoy.

Chard Surprise

Vegan ∘ Serves 2 ∘ Gluten Free

1 Bunch Chard, Thinly Sliced

2 Plums, Pitted And Diced

1 Cup Blueberries

½ Cup Sunflower Seeds

1 Carrot, Shredded

1 Lemon, Juiced

1 Teaspoon Herbamare

1. Thinly Slice The Chard, Including The Stems. Place In A Large Mixing Bowl.
2. Dice The Plums And Shred The Carrot. Add To Chard.
3. Place Sunflower Seeds On Top Of Chard Along With Herbamare.
4. Drizzle Lemon Juice Over Ingredients And Lightly Massage 2-3 Minutes To Incorporate Seasonings.
5. Add Blueberries And Toss To Combine.

Fiesta Salad

Vegan ○ Serves 2 ○ Gluten Free

12 Oz. Shredded Cabbage

1 Small Carrot, Shredded

1 Small Green Bell Pepper, Fine Dice

1 Small Beet, Finely Dice

¼ Small Red Onion, Fine Dice

½ Bunch Cilantro, Chopped

1 Small Jalapeno, Finely Dice

1 Lime, Juiced

1 Tablespoon Herbamare

1 Teaspoon Raw Agave Nectar

1. Prepare All Veg And Place In Mixing Bowl.
2. Add Seasoning, Juice And Nectar.
3. Toss To Mix And Enjoy.

Grapefruit Salad

Vegan ∘ Serves 2 ∘ Gluten Free

2 Grapefruit, Peeled   1 Bunch Watercress

1 Bunch Parsley

1. Peel And Segment Grapefruit. Place In Bowl.
2. Rough Chop Parsley And Watercress. Add To Grapefruit.
3. Toss Together and Enjoy!

Summer Slaw

Vegan ○ Serves 2 ○ Gluten Free

3 Small Yellow Squash,
Shredded

2 Small Carrots,
Shredded

½ Small Red Onion,
Finely Dice

½ Cup Sunflower Seeds,
Soaked

½ Cup Pumpkin Seeds,
Soaked

2 Teaspoons
Herbamare

1 Lemon, Juiced

1. Soak Sunflower Seeds And Pumpkin Seeds Separately Under 1-Inch Purified Water For 2 Hours. Drain And Rinse.

2. Prep All Veg And Place In Mixing Bowl. Add Seeds.

3. Add Juice And Herbamare, Toss To Mix.

4. This Dish Is Great By Itself Or Over Spring Mix Or Baby Spinach.

Fall Festival Salad

Vegan ○ Serves 4 ○ Gluten Free

2 Medium Honeycrisp
  Apples

2 Green Plums

1 Red Pear

1 Small Bunch Mint

1 Lemon, Juiced

1. Wash All Fruit And Mint.
2. Small Dice All Fruit And Place In Bowl.
3. Chiffonade Mint And Place In Bowl.
4. Pour Lemon Juice Over Fruit, Toss And Enjoy.

Avocado Something

Vegan ∘ Serves 2 ∘ Gluten Free

1 Avocado, Diced

1 Peach, Diced

2-3 Green Onions, Sliced

½ Cucumber, Seeded, Diced

1 Jalapeno, Seeded, Minced

1/3 Bunch Cilantro, Chopped

1 Lime, Juiced

1. Prep All Produce And Put Into Medium Mixing Bowl.
2. Add Lime Juice, Toss Gently And Serve.

Mango Lotta Flavor

Vegan ○ Serves 2 ○ Gluten Free

1 Mango, Peeled And Diced

1 Red Pepper, 1" Dice

1/3 Bunch, Cilantro, Chopped

1 Jalapeno, Seeded And Minced

1 Lime, Juiced

½ Cup Raw Pumpkin Seeds

1. Prep All Produce And Place In Medium Bowl.
2. Toss With Pumpkin Seeds And Lime Juice. Enjoy.

Kiwi Plum

Vegan ◦ Serves 2 ◦ Gluten Free

2 Kiwi, Peeled And
  Diced

1 Yellow Pepper, Diced

1-2 Purple Plums, Diced

½ Bunch Cilantro,
  Chopped

1 Lime, Juiced

1. Wash And Prep All Veg And Fruit.

2. Put Into Mixing Bowl, Pour Lime Juice Over All
   Produce. You May Add Minced Fresh Jalapenos
   Or Crushed Red Pepper For Spice.

3. Toss And Serve By Itself Or Over Spring Mix.

Hot In The City

Vegan ○ Serves 2 ○ Gluten Free

1 Navel Orange, Peeled With A Knife And Cut Into Segments, Reserve Juice

1 Green Bell Pepper, Diced

1 Mango, Peeled And Diced

1 Red Bell Pepper, Diced

1 Jalapeno Pepper, Seeded And Diced – Beware Of How Spicy It Is

½ Bunch Flat Parsley, Chopped (Or Cilantro)

1 Lime Juiced, Optional

1. Prep All Fruit And Veg.
2. Put All Into Medium Mixing Bowl. Add Reserved Orange Juice.
3. Toss And Enjoy.

This Recipe Is Great By Itself, Over Spinach Or With Shrimp Or Chicken (Step 3).

Jicama Orange Cilantro

Vegan ∘ Serves 2 ∘ Gluten Free

1 Medium Jicama, Peeled And Julienned

1 Orange, Peeled And Cut In Wedges

1 Red Bell Pepper, Small Dice

1 Jalapeno, Seeded And Minced

½ Bunch Cilantro, Chopped

1 Lime, Juiced

Sea Salt, To Taste

1. Peel Jicama And Julienne. Place Into A Medium Bowl.

2. Peel Orange With Paring Knife And Cut Into Wedges. Reserve Juice. Add To Jicama.

3. Prep Both Peppers And Add To Jicama, Orange Combo.

4. Season With Sea Salt, Lime And Orange Juices. Toss To Combine.

5. You May Let It Sit 30 Minutes For Flavors To Combine Or Eat After It Is Made.

Summer Refresher

Vegan ○ Serves 2 ○ Gluten Free

1 Large Cucumber, Seeded And Small Chop

4 Roma Tomatoes, Small Chop

1 Small Red Onion, Thin Slice

½ Bunch Mint, Chopped

1 Bunch Parsley, Rough Chop

1 Lemon, Juiced

1 Teaspoon Sea Salt

1 Teaspoon Black Pepper

1. Prep All Veg And Put In Medium Bowl.

2. Juice Lemon And Drizzle Over Veggies. Follow With Salt And Pepper.

3. Stir To Combine And Indulge.

Kale, Berry Orange

Vegan ∘ Serves 2 ∘ Gluten Free

1 Bunch Kale, Chopped

1 Cup Fresh Berries

1 Orange, Peeled And Cut Into Wedges

½ Red Onion, Thinly Slice

½ Cup Sunflower Seeds

½ Cup Shredded Coconut

2 Tablespoons Coconut Aminos

1 Teaspoon Herbamare

1. Chop Kale Into Bite-Sized Pieces And Put Into Large Bowl.

2. Cut Onion And Add.

3. Peel Orange With A Paring Knife, Then Cut Out The Segments, Following The Nature Of The Fruit. Squeeze In Any Remaining Juice.

4. Add Sunflower Seeds, And Coconut Aminos.

5. Massage Kale Mixture With Hands For 2 Minutes, To Get The Flavors Into The Leaves.

6. Add Berries On Top Of Kale; If Using Strawberries, Cut Off Ends And Slice. Toss Once More To Mix.

Watermelon Cucumber

Vegan ○ Serves 4 ○ Gluten Free

3 Cups Watermelon, Cut Bite-Sized

1 Medium Cucumber, Seeded, Small Dice

1 Avocado, Small Dice

1 Small Shallot, Minced

2 Teaspoon Mint, Chiffonade

1 Lime, Juiced

1 Sm Bag Spinach Arugula, Chopped

Sea Salt And Pepper To Taste

1. Cut Watermelon Cubes Into Bite Sized Pieces. Place In Medium Bowl.

2. Cut Ends Off Cucumber, Slice In Half Lengthwise And Remove Seeds With A Teaspoon. Cut Into ½ Inch Strips And Dice. Add To Watermelon.

3. Cut Avocado In Half And Remove Pit With A Paring Knife. Cut Into Squares While Still In The Skin. Remove With Teaspoon And Add To Bowl.

4. Thinly Slice (Chiffonade) Mint And Add. Rough Chop Spinach/Arugula Mix And Place On Top Of Fruit/Veggie Mix.

5. Juice The Lime, Pour On Top And Toss To Mix. Season To Taste.

Tropical Chop

Vegan ○ Serves 2 ○ Gluten Free

1 Mango, Peeled And Diced

1 Avocado, Diced

1 Red Bell Pepper, Small Dice

1 Medium Cucumber, Seeded And Diced

2 Tsp Mint, Chiffonade

1 Lime, Juiced

1 Tsp Ground Cumin

1 Bag Baby Spinach

Herbamare, To Taste

1. Slice Mango Along Pit On Both Sides. Cut Into Squares While Still In Skin And Then Slice Out, Into A Medium Bowl. Do The Same With The Avocado.

2. Cut Ends Off Cucumber, Slice In Half Lengthwise And Remove Seeds With A Teaspoon. Cut Into ½-Inch Strips And Dice.

3. Prep Red Pepper Add To Bowl, Along With Chiffonade Mint.

4. Sprinkle Spinach Over Ingredients, Add Seasonings And Lime Juice. Toss To Combine.

Zucchini, Fennel, Tomato Salad

Vegan ○ Serves 2 ○ Gluten Free

1 Small Zucchini, Small Dice

2 Tablespoons Fresh Basil, Chopped

1 Bulb Fennel

1 Lemon, Juiced

1 Medium Tomato, Chopped

2 Teaspoons Herbamare

1. Prep All Veg And Place In Medium Bowl.
2. Toss With Lemon And Basil. Season To Taste With Herbamare.

Vocabulary

Hot Dishes

Mediterranean Stir Fry

Vegan ○ Serves 2 ○ Gluten Free

1 Large Can Garbanzo Beans, Drained

1 Medium Zucchini, Medium Dice

1 Small Tomato, Medium Dice

1 Tablespoon Olive Oil

1 Teaspoon Ground Cumin

2 Teaspoon Oregano

1 Teaspoon Turmeric

3 Cloves Garlic, Mince Herbamare

1. Prepare All Veg And Garlic; Keep Garlic Separate.

2. In Sauté Pan, Heat Olive Oil. When Hot To Touch, Add Garlic, Oregano, Cumin And Turmeric, Toast 2 Minutes. Add Garbanzo And Veg. Sauté Until Zucchini Is Tender 5-10 Minutes.

3. Season With Herbamare To Taste.

Adapted From Hain Recipe

Sweet Potato No Tomato Chili

Vegan ∘ Serves 2 ∘ Gluten Free

1 Large Or 2 Medium Sweet Potatoes, Peeled And Small Dice

1 Small Onion, Small Dice

1 Small Zucchini, Med Dice

1 Small Yellow Squash, Med Dice

1 Small Red Pepper, Med Dice

1 Clove Garlic, Minced

1 Teaspoon Ground Cumin

1 Tablespoon Chili Powder

½ Teaspoon Crushed Red Pepper

¼ Teaspoon White Pepper

1 Tablespoon Olive Oil

1. Prep All Veg.

2. Put Sauce Pot On Medium High With Olive Oil. When Oil Is Hot (1-2 Minutes) Add Garlic, Onions, Crushed Red Pepper. Lightly Toast.

3. When Onions Are Shiny Add All Other Veggies And Spices. Stir Together And Cook 2 -3 Minutes.

4. Add ¼ Cup Water, Reduce Heat To Medium, Cover And Cook 20 Minutes, Until Veggies Are Soft.

5. Season To Taste With Herbamare Or Sea Salt.

(You May Add ½ Meat – Ground Beef, Turkey Or Cut Up Chicken To This At Time Of Adding Veggies)

Asparagus, Zucchini, And Tomato

Vegan ∘ Serves 2 ∘ Gluten Free

1 Bunch Asparagus, Chopped Into 1-Inch Pieces

3 Cloves Garlic, Minced

1 Large Zucchini, Small Dice

Sea Salt, To Taste

1 Large Tomato, Diced

1 Lemon, Juiced

½ Bunch Cilantro, Chopped

1. Prep And Steam Zucchini And Asparagus. Let Cool.

2. Toss With Other Ingredients. Or Toss Together While Hot and Serve.

Meat, Fish and Seafood

Chicken Tabouli

Serves 1 ○ Gluten Free

1 Sm Bag Spring Mix Or Baby Spinach, Or 2 Bunches Parsley

1 Small Red Onion, Small Dice

3 ½ Oz. Chicken, Steamed And Chopped

1 Clove Garlic, Minced

1 Small Tomato, Diced

1 Lemon, Juiced

Sea Salt To Taste

1. Rough Chop Spring Mix, Spinach, Or Parsley.
2. Chop Chicken Into Small Pieces.
3. Toss Chicken With Greens, Tomato, Garlic, And Onion.
4. Season With Lemon Juice And Salt.

Stuffed Zucchini

Serves 1 ∘ Gluten Free

1 Medium Zucchini

3 ½ Oz. Fish, Shrimp,
Or Chicken, Cut Into
Small Cubes

1 Small Tomato, Small
Dice

1 Teaspoon Garlic Salt

1 Teaspoon Italian
Herbs

1. Fill Pot With 3 Inches Water And Put Steamer On Top.

2. Slice Zucchini In Half Lengthwise And Scoop Out Seeds With Teaspoon.

3. When Steamer Is Hot, Place Zucchini In, Scooped Side Down, For 6 Minutes. Take Out And Let Cool.

4. While Zucchini Is Cooling, In Water Left In Pot, Sauté Tomato, Protein, Garlic Salt And Herbs Until Cooked, About 5-7 Minutes.

5. Pour Into Zucchini Boats And Enjoy.

Option – *Try 1 Drained Can Of White Beans In Place Of The Meat/Fish/Shrimp.*

Shrimp & Spinach Saute

Serves 1 ○ Gluten Free

6 Shrimp

½ Red Bell Pepper
Thinly Slice

1 Small Bag Spinach

1 Clove Garlic

½ Small Red Onion
Thinly Sliced

Olive Oil

Chicken Broth

Sea Salt

Black Pepper

1. Toast Garlic In Olive Oil Add Red Pepper And Red Onion. Add Shrimp.
2. Add Spinach And Cover Until Only Wilted. Deglaze With Chicken Broth. Season With Sea Salt And Pepper.

Option – *Drained White Beans Or Garbanzo Beans Make A Great Substitute.*

Salmon, Potato, Artichoke

Serves 2 ° Gluten Free

8 Oz. Wild Salmon Fillet, Cut In Half, Skin Off

8 Oz. Veggie Or Chicken Broth

2 Small/1 Large Yukon Gold Potatoes, Thinly Sliced 1-15 Oz. Can Artichoke Hearts, Quartered, Drained

Herbamare To Taste

1. Preheat Oven To 425 Degrees.

2. Add 40 Oz. Broth To 10-Inch Sauté Pan And Bring To Boil. Add Potatoes In An Even Layer In Bottom Of Pan. Reduce To Simmer And Cook 5 -7 Minutes Until Potatoes Are Tender.

3. Add Salmon On Top Of Potatoes And Then Layer The Artichoke Hearts Around The Fish And In Between The 2 Fillets, On Top Of The Potatoes.

4. Add Remaining Broth, Cover With Lid, And Place In Oven For 12 -15 Minutes.

5. Season To Taste With Herbamare And Enjoy.

Kale, Sweet Potato, Sausage Stew

Serves 2 ○ Gluten Free

2 Links Turkey Sausage

1 Bunch Dinosaur Kale, Chopped

1 Red Onion, Small Dice

1 Medium Sweet Potato, Peeled And Diced

1 -14.5oz Can Fire-Roasted Tomatoes

1 Tablespoon Olive Oil

1 Teaspoon Each: Paprika, Turmeric, And Cumin

Sea Salt, Black Pepper

1. Prep All Veg.

2. In Stock Pot, Heat Olive Oil On Med High Heat. Sauté Onion And Sweet Potato For 5 Minutes. Add Sausage, Out Of Its Casing. Sauté Until It Begins To Brown.

3. Add Kale, Spices And ½ Cup Water. Stir To Combine, Scraping Any Browned Bits From Bottom Of Pot.

4. Add Tomatoes, Stir And Reduce Heat To Medium Once Stew Comes To A Boil, Cover And Cook 15 Minutes, Until Potatoes Are Soft.

Chicken, Spinach, Tomato, Walnut

Serves 2 ○ Gluten Free

6-8 Oz. Chicken Breast Or Tenders

1 Large Or 2 Small Bags Baby Spinach

2 Roma Tomatoes, Small Dice

3 Cloves Garlic, Minced

3 Tablespoons Chopped Walnuts

Olive Oil

Herbamare

Chicken Stock Or Water

1. Mince Garlic And Dice Tomato.

2. Season Chicken With Herbamare On Both Sides.

3. Place 2 Teaspoons Olive Oil In Sauté Pan And Heat On Medium High. When Hot, Add Chicken And Sauté 5- 7 Minutes.

4. Turn Over, Add Garlic, Spinach And ¼ Cup Broth Or Water. Cover And Cook 3-5 Minutes.

5. Stir, Add Tomatoes And Walnuts. Cook 2 -3 Minutes Until The Moisture Is Cooked Off.

Beef Stuffed Eggplant

Serves 2 • Gluten Free

1 Medium Eggplant

1/2 Pound Ground Beef

1 Small Onion, Diced

2 Roma Tomato, Small Dice

1 Clove Garlic, Minced

1 Teaspoon Oregano

½ Bag French-Cut Green Beans

½ Teaspoon Sea Salt

Olive Oil

1. Preheat Oven 425.

2. Make 6 Punctures In Eggplant With Fork And Place In Oven On Middle Rack. Bake 25 Minutes. Remove And Let Cool Slightly.

3. While Eggplant Is Cooking, Sauté Garlic And Onion In A Medium Sauté Pan With Olive Oil Until Onions Are Shiny. Add Ground Beef And Cook Thoroughly. Season With Oregano And Sea Salt.

4. When Eggplant Is Cool Enough To Touch, Cut In Half And Cut Out Middle. Cut Into Small Dice And Add To Beef Mixture, Along With Tomato And Green Beans.

5. Cook Together 2-3 Minutes To Blend All Flavors. Spoon Into Eggplant Shells And Warm In Oven For 5 -7 Minutes.

Option – I Like To Sauté A Large Portobello Mushroom, Thinly Sliced, Or 6 -8 Baby Bella Mushrooms, Sliced, In Place Of The Meat.

Zone Fish

Serves 2 ∘ Gluten Free

2 - 6oz Fillets Cod

1 - 15oz Can Fire
Roasted Tomatoes

½ Bag French Cut Green
Beans

Herbamare

1. Preheat Oven To 425.

2. In Square Baking Pan Place Fish, Then Green
   Beans, Tomatoes And Season With Herbamare.

3. Cover With Parchment Paper Or Foil And Cook
   25 Minutes.

Adapted From Zone Recipes

Chicken, Roasted Tomato and Artichoke

Serves 2 ○ Gluten Free

1/2 Pounds Chicken Tenders

1 - 14oz Can Fire Roasted Tomatoes

1 -14 Oz. Can Artichoke Heart Quarters

1 Teaspoon Oregano

2 Teaspoon Herbamare

1 Teaspoon Olive Oil

1. Heat Olive Oil In Sauté Pan Over Medium-High Heat.

2. Add Chicken, Season With Herbamare. When Cooked Halfway Through, Turn Over And Place Artichoke Hearts Around The Chicken. Pour Roasted Tomatoes Over The Artichokes And Chicken And Season With Oregano.

3. Reduce To Simmer, Cover And Cook 6 -8 Minutes Until Chicken Is Cooked.

Option – *For Me It Is The Northern Bean Or Cannelini That Make This A Great Plant-Based Dish.*

Pizza Soup

Serves 2 ∘ Gluten Free

Olive Oil

2 Italian Sausage Links

Half-Bag Frozen Chopped Broccoli

3 Cups Broth

14.5 Oz. Can Chopped Fire-Roasted Tomatoes

2-3 Teaspoons Pizza Seasoning/Italian Seasoning

1. Heat Some Olive Oil In A Sauté Pan, Remove Sausage From Casing And Brown The Sausage.

2. Add The Canned Tomatoes And The Pizza Seasoning. Stir To Combine.

3. Pour In The Broth, And Then Add The Broccoli. It Can Be Frozen Or Defrosted; Doesn't Matter.

4. Bring To A Boil, And Then Simmer For 10 Minutes.

Chopped Steak Tabouli

Serves 2 ∘ Gluten Free

1 Large Bag Baby Spinach

12oz New York Strip Steak.

1 Small Plum Tomato

Juice Of ½ Lemon

2 Tablespoons Olive Oil

1 Teaspoon Sea Salt

1 Teaspoon Granulated Garlic

1. Season Steak With Salt And Pepper, Sear Steak To Desired Temperature And Cool In Refrigerator.
2. Chop Baby Spinach And Place In Bowl. Dice Tomato And Add To Spinach.
3. Dice Steak; Add To Mixture.
4. Whisk Dressing Ingredients Together And Pour Over When Ready To Serve.

Steamed Grouper With Asparagus, Zucchini And Tomato

Serves 2 ∘ Gluten Free

8 Oz. Grouper Fillet/ Other Meaty White Fish

Seasoning of Choice

1 Bunch Asparagus, Chopped 1-Inch Pieces

3 Cloves Garlic, Minced

1 Large Zucchini, Small Dice

Sea Salt, To Taste

1 Large Tomato, Diced

1 Lemon, Juiced

½ Bunch Cilantro, Chopped

1. Get Steamer Ready.
2. Sprinkle Seasoning On Grouper.
3. Place Grouper In Top Steamer Pan. Steam 5 Minutes.
4. Prep Zucchini And Asparagus And Place With Garlic In Tray Under Grouper. Continue To Steam 5 – 8 More Minutes.
5. Toss Veg With Other Ingredients.
6. Serve With Lemon Wedges.

Pygmalion

We are at your final destination! These recipes take you to the finish line and beyond. Now you get to add back those final food triggers and see what makes you gain weight, makes you bloated, what you may allow back into your eating lifestyle and what you may have on occasion. Here are the recipes that will keep you on track and still enjoy your life. The nice part is that you get to mix all the recipes together now. You are now graduating with the knowledge of your "real language of food" to live your healthiest life and beyond.

Pygmalion

Soups

Beans, Greens And Grains

Vegan ○ Serves 2 ○ Gluten Free

1 Bunch Kale, Chard Or Collards

2 Medium Carrots, Diced Small

1 Stalk Celery, Fine Diced

1 Small Yellow Onion, Finely Diced

½ Cup Quinoa

½ Cup Lentils

1 Tablespoon Herbamare

2 Tablespoons Granulated Garlic

2 Teaspoons Powdered Onion

1. Prepare All Veg And Place In Stockpot, Cover With 6 Cups Of Water. Place On Burner, Bring To Boil.

2. Add Quinoa, Lentils, And Spices.

3. Bring Back To Boil, Reduce To Simmer, Cover And Cook 45 Minutes.

4. Enjoy.

Detox Friendly: *Leave Out Carrots And Grains*

Pygmalion

Cold Dishes

Quinoa Surprise

Vegan ○ Serves 4 ○ Gluten Free

1 Cup Quinoa

½ Bag Edamame

1 Small Red Onion, Finely Diced

1 Stalk Celery, Finely Diced

1/2 Cup Raw Pumpkin Seeds

Dressing

1/3 Cup Coconut Aminos

1/3 Cup Balsamic Vinegar

1/4 Cup Olive Oil

2 Teaspoons Italian Herbs

1. Bring 2 Cups Of Water To A Boil In Sauce Pot With 1 Cup Quinoa. Reduce To Simmer And Cook Until Liquid Is Absorbed (15- 20 Minutes).

   Remove From Burner, Add Frozen Edamame, And Stir Together. Pour Into Bowl And Refrigerate Until Cool, Approximately 20-30 Minutes.

2. While Quinoa Is Cooling, Prepare Veg. Combine Dressing Ingredients In Separate Bowl And Whisk Together.

3. When Quinoa Is Cool, Combine All Ingredients, Pour Dressing Over, Toss To Combine And Enjoy.

Tabouli, Adrienne Style

Vegan ∘ Serves 2 ∘ Gluten Free

1sm Bag Spring Mix Or Baby Spinach, Rough Chop

1 Small Red Onion, Finely Diced

1 Small Tomato, Dice

1/3 Cup Quinoa, Uncooked

1/3 Cup Lemon Juice

1/4 Cup Olive Oil

1 Teaspoon Sea Salt

2 Teaspoons Granulated Garlic

1. In Small Saucepot, Bring 2/3 Cup Water And Quinoa To Boil. Reduce To Simmer And Cook 15 Minutes, Until Liquid Is Absorbed. Refrigerate To Cool.

2. While Quinoa Is Cooling, Prepare All Veggies And Place In One Bowl.

3. Prepare Dressing In Separate Bowl And Whisk Together, Set Aside.

4. When Quinoa Is Cooled, Pour Over Veg. Drizzle Dressing Over Tabouli And Toss To Combine.

5. Serve As Is Or Chill 20 Minutes.

Wild Rice And Cranberry

Vegan ∘ Serves 4 ∘ Gluten Free

1 Bag Frozen Wild Rice Blend (Defrosted)

3 Stalks Organic Celery, Diced

1/2 Cup Dried Organic Cranberries

1/3 Cup Walnut Pieces, Soaked

1 /2 Cup Pumpkin Seeds

3 Green Onions, Chopped

1. Take Rice Out Of Freezer The Night Before And Place In Refrigerator To Defrost.
2. Place Walnuts In Bowl With 1 Cup Of Water And Soak In Refrigerator Overnight.
3. Chop Celery And Place In Medium Bowl. Add Rice, Cranberries, Pumpkin Seeds And Drained Walnut Pieces.
4. Mix, Season To Taste With Sea Salt And Pepper. Serve.

Quinoa, Avocado, Spinach

Vegan ○ Serves 2 ○ Gluten Free

1/3 Cup Uncooked Quinoa

1/2 Avocado, Diced

1 Small Shallot, Finely Diced

1 Small Zucchini, Grated

1 Small Carrot, Grated

1 Bag Baby Spinach

1 Lemon, Juiced

1 - 2 Teaspoons Sea Salt

1/2 Teaspoon White Pepper

1 Tsp Herbamare

1. Bring To Boil In Small Saucepot, 2/3 Cup Water And Quinoa. Reduce To Simmer And Cook 15 -20 Minutes Until All Liquid Is Absorbed. Remove From Pot And Let Cool Completely In Refrigerator.

2. While Quinoa Is Cooking/Cooling, Prep All Veg. You May Rough Chop Spinach If You Like And Add To Mix.

3. When Quinoa Is Cooled, Add To Veggies Along With Lemon Juice And Seasonings. Toss To Mix.

4. Season To Taste.

Quinoa Confetti

Vegan ○ Serves 4 ○ Gluten Free

1 Cup Uncooked Quinoa

1 Raw Broccoli Crown

1 Small Carrot, Fine Dice

1 Small Red Pepper, Fine Diced

½ Medium Red Onion, Fine Diced

1 Small Green Pepper, Fine Diced

1 Lemon, Juiced

2 Tablespoons Olive Oil

1 Teaspoon Sea Salt

½ Teaspoon Black Pepper

1. Cook Quinoa In 2 Cups Water In Sauce Pot. Bring To A Boil, Reduce To Simmer And Cook 15 Minutes, Until Liquid Is Absorbed. Place On A Plate And Let Cool Completely In Refrigerator.

2. While Quinoa Is Cooking/Cooling, Remove All Florets From Broccoli With Paring Knife. Prep All Other Veg, And Place In Mixing Bowl.

3. When Quinoa Is Completely Cooled, Place In Bowl With Other Veg.

4. In Small Mixing Bowl, Mix Together The Lemon Juice, Salt, Pepper And Olive Oil.

5. Pour Over Quinoa And Veg And Mix Together.

6. You May Let It Rest For 15 Minutes Or Enjoy As Is.

Pygmalion

Hot Dishes

Amaranth Stuffed Zucchini

Vegan ○ Serves 2 ○ Gluten Free

2 Medium Zucchini, Cut In Half Lengthwise

1 -2 Roma Tomato, Small Dice

½ Cup Amaranth, Uncooked

1 Medium Yellow Onion, Small Dice

4 -6 Cremini Or Baby Bella Mushrooms, Thinly Sliced

Olive Oil

Herbamare

Sea Salt

1. Preheat Oven To 425 Degrees. Place 1 ½ Cups Water And ½ Cup Amaranth In Sauce Pot And Bring To Boil. Lower To Simmer, Cover And Cook 20 – 30 Minutes, Until Liquid Is Absorbed. Remove From Heat And Stir.

2. Slice Zuke In Half Lengthwise, And Scoop Seeds Out With Teaspoon Or Melon Scoop, Being Careful Not To Break Bottom Or Sides Of Squash.

3. Lightly Coat Squash With Olive Oil And Sprinkle With Herbamare. Place On Cookie Sheet And Bake For 12 -15 Minutes.

4. Heat Sauté Pan Over Medium High, Add Oil And Onions, And Sprinkle With Sea Salt. Cook Until Slightly Caramelized, Approximately 10 -15 Minutes.

5. While Onions Are Caramelizing, Chop Zuke Centers, Slice Mushroom And Dice Tomato. Add Zuke And Mushroom To Onion. Sauté 7 -10 Minutes. Remove From Heat.

6. Remove Zuke Shells From Oven. Add Tomato And Amaranth To Zuke Mixture In Sauté Pan. Season With Herbamare And Mix Together. Spoon Into Shells.

7. Put Back In Oven 3 -5 Minutes.

8. You May Add Goat Cheese Or Cheese Of Choice At End And Meat In Oven Also.

Butternut Quinoa

Vegan ∘ Serves 2 ∘ Gluten Free

2-3 Cup Diced Butternut Squash

1 Small Onion, Small Dice

1 cup Frozen Peas, Defrosted

1 Small Jar Roasted Red Pepper, Small Dice

½ Cup Dried Cranberries

½ Cup Pumpkin Seeds

¼ Teaspoon Cloves

¼ Teaspoon Nutmeg

1 Teaspoon Cinnamon

1 Teaspoon Sea Salt

1 Tablespoon Olive Oil

1 Cup Quinoa (Uncooked)

1. Boil 2 Cups Water With 1 Cup Quinoa. Bring To Simmer, Cook 10-12 Minutes Until Liquid Is Absorbed. Place In Medium/Large Serving Bowl.

2. Prep All Veg And Have Ready At Stove To Add To Cooking.

3. In Large Sauté Pan, Heat Olive Oil Over Medium High Heat. Add Onion And A Little Sea Salt. Sauté Until Onions Are Shiny.

4. When Onions Are Shiny, Add Spices, Then Squash And Sea Salt. Add 1/4 -1/2 Cup Of Water, Stir And Cover. Cook 8-12 Minutes, Until Squash Is Soft.

5. When Squash Is Cooked, Add To Quinoa, Along With Peas, Peppers, Cranberries And Pumpkin Seeds.

6. Adjusted Seasonings To Taste.

   If Using Frozen Squash, Then Cook To Only Heat Squash Through And Continue With Rest Of Recipe.

Mojadara

Vegan ∘ Serves 4 ∘ Gluten Free

1 Cup Dry Lentils

1 ½ Cups Brown
Basmati Rice

1 Large Yellow Onion,
Thinly Sliced

1 Tablespoon Ground
Cumin

Olive Oil

Sea Salt

1. Boil 3 Cups Of Water, Add Lentils. Bring Back To Boil, Reduce To Simmer. Cook 20 Minutes. Drain Lentils, Reserving Water From Lentils To Cook Rice In. Season With Cumin.

2. Combine Lentil-Reserved Water With Enough Extra Water To Make 3 Cups Water. In Same Pot As Lentils Were Cooked In, Bring Water To Boil, Add Rice, Bring Back To Boil, Reduce To Simmer, Cover And Cook 30-45 Minutes Until Water Is Absorbed.

3. Pour Rice Over Lentils And Sprinkle With 2 Teaspoons Sea Salt. Do Not Stir Together Yet.

4. While Rice Is Cooking, Place Onions In Small Sauté Pan. Sprinkle With 1 Teaspoon Sea Salt And Drizzle Onions With Olive Oil To Cover Them All. Caramelize Over Medium Low Heat Until All Onions Are Golden Brown, Stirring Occasionally.

This Cooking Process Will Take 20 Minutes, At Least. The Onions Will Cook Unevenly, So Keep An Eye On Them To Prevent Burning.

5. Pour Over Rice When Onions Are Cooked. Stir All Ingredients Now And Season To Taste With More Cumin Or Sea Salt, If Needed.

Veggie Lasagna

Serves 4-6 ∘ Gluten Free

1 Box Tinkayada Lasagna

1 Box Frozen Butternut Squash

1 -12 Oz Jar Rst Red Peppers

1 Lb Portobella Mushrooms

2 Boxes Frozen Spinach

1- 24 Oz. Jar Newman's Own Organic Pasta Sauce

Olive Oil

Herbamare

. . . .

Put Froz Veg In Fridge To Defrost The Day Before Making

1. Preheat Oven 425 Degrees.
2. Precook Pasta According To Instructions. Reduce Cooking Time By 3 Minutes.
3. Remove Gills Of Mushrooms (Black Part With A Teaspoon) Slice Thin, Season With Herbmare Or Sea Salt And Pepper, And Sauté Until Tender.
4. Drain Spinach By Squeezing All Excess Water By Hand.
5. In 13 X 9" Pan, Place Thin Layer Of Sauce.
6. Lay Out 3 Noodles. Place Thin Layer Of Butternut Squash, Spinach, And Mushrooms.

7. Cover With Thin Layer Of Sauce And Place 3 Noodles On Top.

8. Spread Thin Layer Of Squash Followed By Spinach, And Roasted Peppers.

9. Cover With Sauce And Last Layer Of Noodles.

10. Cover With Remaining Sauce. Add Enough Water To Fill Pan Halfway. Cover And Bake 35 -45 Minutes.

11. Remove From Oven, Remove Cover And Let Set 15 Minutes Before Serving.

Pasta Artichoke

Serves 2 ○ Gluten Free

1/2 Bag Tinkyada Penne Pasta

1-15oz Can Artichoke Heart Quarters

1-6 Oz. Jar Roasted Red Peppers

8-12 Kalamata Pitted Olives

3 Oz. Goat Cheese, Chevre

1 Tablespoon Italian Herbs

Herbamare

Olive Oil

1. Cook Pasta 8 -15 Minutes, Until Al Dente (Package Times Are Off, So Start Checking Doneness After 8 Minutes). Drain And Rinse. Pasta May Be Held For Later Use Or Continue With Recipe.

2. Drain Artichoke Hearts, Roasted Red Peppers And Olives. Slice Olives For More Flavor, If Preferred.

3. Slice Roasted Red Peppers, If They Are Not Already.

4. Place Pasta In Large Bowl And Add Other Ingredients. Finish With A Drizzle Of Olive Oil.

5. Season With Herbamare.

Manchego Mushrooms

Serves 2 ∘ Gluten Free

1 Small Container Baby
Bella Mushrooms

4 Oz. Manchego Cheese

Olive Oil

Sea Salt

Black Pepper

1. Preheat Oven To Broil.
2. Thickly Slice Mushrooms And Place On Cookie Sheet.
3. Drizzle With Olive Oil, Salt, And Pepper.
4. Thinly Slice Or Shred On Grater Manchego And Place Over Mushrooms.
5. Place Under Broiler On Second To Top Rack, Until Cheese Is Melted.

Penne, Arugala, Capers, Olives

Serves 2 ○ Gluten Free

½ Bag Tinkayada Penne

1- 6oz. Bag Arugula Or Spinach/Arugula Mix

3 Cloves Garlic, Minced

2 Tablespoons Capers

6 Pitted Kalamata Olives Or Green Olives

Olive Oil

Crushed Red Pepper

Goat Cheese (Step3)

Sea Salt

Black Pepper

1. Boil Water For Pasta With 1 Teaspoon Sea Salt. Add Pasta And Cook 8 – 15 Minutes, Until Tender. Drain And Hold

2. While Pasta Is Cooking, Mince Garlic On Top Of ½ Teaspoon Sea Salt And A Dash Crushed Red Pepper.

3. Heat 1 Tablespoon Olive Oil In Large Sauté Pan, Add Garlic. Toast 30 Seconds. When Aromatic, Add Arugula And Stir With Fork. When Wilted, Add Capers And Olives.

4. Add Pasta To Pan, Toss And Put In Medium Bowl. Season With Salt And Pepper. Add Cheese, If Desired.

Spaghetti Squash W/Spinach

Serves 2 ∘ Gluten Free

1 Sm Spaghetti Squash, Cut In Half	2 -4 Oz. Goat Cheese, Or Romano
1 Bag Baby Spinach	Olive Oil
1 Roma Tomato, Sm Dice	Herbamare
1-3 Cloves Garlic, Minced	Crushed Red Pepper (Optional)

1. Preheat Oven To 425 Degrees. Cut Squash In Half, Place In Pan, Add 1 Inch Water And Place In Oven 30 -45 Minutes, Until Soft To Touch. Remove From Oven, Let Cool Until Able To Hold.

2. When Squash Is Able To Be Held (By Hand Or With A Towel, Scoop Out Seeds. Then With A Fork, Scrape The Squash Out, Separating The Threads Of Spaghetti. Place In Medium Bowl.

3. In A Sauté Pan, Toast Garlic And Crushed Red Pepper In Oil Over Medium High Heat, Until Aromatic.

4. Add Spinach And Sauté Until Wilted, 2 -3 Minutes. Stir Once Or Twice.

5. Add To Squash, Along With Tomato And Cheese. Season To Taste With Herbamare.

Meat, Fish And Seafood

Shrimp Feta Spin

Serves 2 ○ Gluten Free

2/3 Pound Shrimp

½ Small Red Onion Thinly Sliced

1 Clove Garlic

1 Red Bell Pepper Thinly Sliced

1 Large Bag Spinach

Olive Oil

Herbamare

1/2 Box Tinkyada Penne

Feta Or Goat Cheese

1. Put Pot On High To Boil Salted Water To Cook Pasta. When Water Boils, Add Pasta And Cook According To Directions. Start Checking Doneness After 8 Minutes.

2. Put Sauté Pan On Medium High Heat.

3. Toast Garlic In Olive Oil, Add Red Pepper And Red Onion. Add Shrimp And Stir.

4. Add Spinach, Stir And Cover. Cook Until Spinach Is Wilted 2-5 Minutes Stirring Occasionally.

5. Toss With Pasta, Top With Cheese.

Zucchini Feta Chicken

Serves 2 ○ Gluten Free

1/2 Pound Chicken Tenders Or Boneless Chicken Thighs

4 Oz. Feta

2 Zucchini, Sliced In Half Moons

1 Tablespoon Oregano

Olive Oil

2 Teaspoons Herbamare

1. Preheat Oven To 425.

2. Prep Zucchini. Place Chicken In Oven Baking Dish. Place Zucchini Around Chicken. Drizzle Olive Oil Over Meat And Veg. Season With Oregano And Herbamare.

3. Bake 20 Minutes (30 If Using Thighs), Add Feta And Bake Additional 8-10 Minutes Until Cheese Is Melted.

Lemon Olive Chicken With Zucchini

Serves 2 ∘ Gluten Free

1/2 Pound Chicken Tenders

6 Pitted Green Olives, Sliced

Juice 1 Lemon

1 Shallot, Diced

2 Medium Zucchini, Cut Into Half Moons

1 Tablespoon Olive Oil

1 ½ Teaspoons Herbamare

1 Tablespoon. Gluten Free Flour/Almond Flour

½ Cup Chicken Stock

1. Mince Shallot And Sauté In Olive Oil 2 Minutes.
2. Dust Chicken With Flour(Optional) And Add To Pan.
3. Add Zucchini And Sauté Until Chicken Is Almost Done.
4. Add Lemon Juice, Chicken Stock And Olives. Cover And Cook Three More Minutes.
5. Season To Taste With Herbamare.

Caper Chicken And Broccoli

Serves 2 ∘ Gluten Free

½ Pound Chicken Tenders

2 Head Broccoli, Cut Off Florets

3 Tablespoons Capers

4 Oz. Goat Mozzarella, Shredded

Olive Oil

Herbamare

1. Preheat Oven To 425.
2. In Pan, Layer Chicken And Broccoli, Overlapping.
3. Drizzle Olive Oil Over Meat And Veg. Sprinkle With Herbamare.
4. Top With Cheese, Cover, Bake 15 – 20 Minutes Until Done.

Sausage Pizza Mushroom

2 Portobella Mushrooms, Cleaned

½ Pound Turkey Sausage

1- 8 Oz. Can Pizza Sauce

4 Oz. Buffalo Mozzarella

Spray Olive Oil

1. Preheat Oven To 425 Degrees.
2. Clean Mushrooms By Removing Stem And Using A Teaspoon To Scrape Gills Off Mushrooms.
3. Place On Sheet Pan. You May Spray Bottom Of Mushrooms With Oil, If Desired.
4. Take Sausage Out Of The Casing And Place Some Inside Each Mushroom.
5. Top With Sauce And 2 Slices Of Cheese Each.
6. Bake For 15 -20 Minutes.

Lessons Learned

So, now that you've worked your way through the program, made changes in your eating lifestyle, how do you feel? Have you noticed foods that work and do not work in your body? My hope is that you have been able to identify various foods that give you gas, bloating, stomach pain, or ones that make you retain water. If so, clearly those are the foods to stay away from; ideally, not forever, but for just a while longer.

Remember Hippocrates said, "Let food be thy medicine and medicine be thy food." Your body will do whatever is natural, normal or necessary to survive. Your body will self-regulate when it comes to food IF YOU LISTEN TO IT. I am not saying ignore doctors. I am not a dietitian. I'm a chef with a knack for making healthy food that is also excellent for your soul.

Integrate, ask questions, play with both food and medicine. Medicine tells you to consider the intake of certain foods. There is a reason for that. Use all the available information to your benefit. Continue to see your physicians because they are experts in their fields. Have you ever considered yourself to be an expert in the field of your body? **The Real Language of Food** is to get you back to listening to what your body is saying. Food is the dialect of your body. Your digestive tract is the interpreter for your health. Your body will let you know what it can and cannot accept. Your job is to learn to listen.

What happens when your body cannot digest food properly? Life takes a very uncomfortable turn. Listen to your body. When you crave protein, it's because you need it. When you eat something and can't digest it one time, it may be a single occurrence. Bad fish happens. But if every time you drink a glass of milk or eat some pasta, your stomach says, "I don't think so," remove that from your eating choices for a while. Acknowledge and address those results. I have given you plenty of options to replace dairy and wheat. No, they are not the same sometimes, but they ARE a way to still enjoy foods you thought you may no longer be able to have. Things change. You may have broken out in hives as a kid when you ate a strawberry but, by age thirty, that didn't happen anymore. You may experience an intolerance for something for a while, but after taking it out of the picture, you may be able to tolerate it later on down the road. What most people do not realize is that a food sensitivity effects your entire body's health and brain function, not just indigestion. Disruption of sleep, brain fog, joint aches and pains, reduced immune function are all part of food antagonists. Honor your body's needs in the moment. Do what it tells you so you can live a more comfortable life now and twenty years from now.

So, what next? 70% of the population will likely go back to the way they ate before they start their new protocol, expecting their health/digestion to stay the way they feel right now. If you were eating and drinking processed/ prepackaged foods before you started and think, "I did my time, now I will celebrate," or "I'm too busy to do this anymore," well, that is where you have done yourself a great disservice. You committed to twelve weeks of a better lifestyle, you are already in it, why stop now?

But, Adrienne, I am bored with the recipes. I found this great recipe on "X" site, but it has foods that do not agree with me.

Email me. This is not a one and done book. This is my way to reach out to you. I didn't do all of this just to sell books, I'm trying to change lives. There are things we can do together to keep you on path.

We can set up online cooking lessons or you can send me the recipes and I will hack through them to make them easier for you. I am given recipes by clients all the time. They want me to prepare these meals for them and they're way too complicated. That is where my MacGyver culinary skills come into play (as my bestie calls it) and I can ninja recipes for you. The same thing applies for traditional family recipes, I can probably hack them for you. Yes, even your grandmother's best stuff.

Do you own a business or are you a decision maker at a company? How about a new and interesting way to have a corporate wellness *Lunch and Learn*? I can present a topic and do a recipe demo, complete with samplings for your company. Look at the statistics on productivity in the workplace. Healthy workers mean more productivity. When you feel good, you're happier. When you're happier, you're more productive at work as well as at home.

Not everyone can cook and that's where I can help. Most people can learn the basic skills. I offer cooking lessons - online, in your home, for your next dinner party, or at your place of business. Give me thirty minutes online and we can have your dinner meal prepared and ready to eat. Give me an hour in your kitchen and I will walk you through three to five recipes to have prepped for the week. It's easy and it's fun.

We eat for nourishment. We eat for energy. We eat for celebration. We eat for comfort. It's time to start eating for positivity vs. stress eating, which stuffs things back down into you. Why would you want to keep something sad or angry in your body? It literally eats you alive (aka leaky gut). Why let food rot inside you because your body cannot digest it? Instead, how about use food to give you energy, life? Why not eat food that lets you flush out the ugly stuff?

Need help with food preparation? I am The Food Whisperer. I will help you find a way to prepare the foods you like that work for your body. Let's work together to make your body the healthiest and happiest it can be.

Email me at afalconegodsell@gmail.com

Find me on Social Media at

- LinkedIn Adrienne Falcone Godsell
- Facebook iamtfw
- Instagram iamthefoodwhisperer
- YouTube Adrienne Falcone Godsell

GLOSSARY

Vegan	No Animal Product, Including Honey.
Wheat Free	Does Not Contain Any Wheat, But May Still Contain Gluten.
Gluten	A Protein Found in Grains That Produces Digestion Issues.
Gluten Free	Does Not Contain Any Gluten Products.
Candida	A Fungus (Yeast) That Shows Up in Various Forms in The Body.
Candida Friendly	Foods That People Who Have Candida Are Able to Consume and Not Have Candida Issues.
Herbamare	An Msg-Free Herb Seasoning, Great For Salads With Olive Oil And A Lemon Wedge, On Veggies, Meat, Fish, Or To Season Soups Instead Of Soup Base.
Italian Herbs	Frontier Makes a Great Italian Herb Mix
Veganaise	An Eggless, Gluten Free, Mayo.

**Quinoa
(Keen-Wa!)**

A Gluten Free Grain That Contains All Essential Amino Acids That Complete A Protein.

Amaranth

A Gluten Free Grain, That Is Very Aromatic. Cooks Up Similar to Sticky Rice.

Xanthan Gum

An Emulsifying Agent Used Also As A Binding Agent In Gluten Free Cooking. May Be Used as A Thickener Also, But If Too Much The Liquid Will Become Gummy.

FUN FOOD FACTS

Black beans - All beans have protease inhibitors, which may inhibit tumor growth. The fiber binds with toxins in the colon and carries them out before they can be reabsorbed. Beans or legumes are a great plant based source of fiber and protein, as well as B complex.

Quinoa – A "Mother Grain," this super food was considered a sacred crop by the Incas. It is the only gluten free grain to have all the essential amino acids that make a complete protein as well as being fiber, calcium and iron rich. It is a great alternative to wheat and gluten-containing grains which can be inflammatory

Pumpkin seeds – Pumpkin seeds have a bioavailable source of vitamin E not readily available in food sources. This type of Vitamin E makes pumpkin seeds a great antioxidant to rid the body of free radicals. They are also rich in zinc and magnesium. A quarter cup of pumpkin seeds has 9.75 grams of protein and 2 grams of fiber. It also contains linoleic acid, and essential fatty acid which the body needs to promote wound healing.

Tomato – Carotene rich foods act as free radical scavengers stimulating the immune system and may even be toxic to tumors. Lycopene is the factor in tomatoes that has anti-cancer properties to it.

Garlic and onion – The allium group of vegetables speed the body's elimination of carcinogens. Garlic and onions have been cultivated for over 5000 years, dating back to Central Asia and the Middle East. Egyptians spent large amounts of money to feed workers meals based on garlic and onions. The allium group protects against nitrosamines found in the intestine formed by nitrites.

Spring mix/spinach – Dark leafy green veggies contain soluble and insoluble fiber, making them important for the cleansing of the colon and production of good bacteria in the gut. They also help keep blood sugar levels stable, 'starving' glucose-hungry cancer cells.

Zucchini – Known as one of the 'three sisters' by Native Americans long with corn and beans, zucchini's skin is particularly rich in antioxidants and its pectin-rich polysaccharide middle has been found to assist the body in better regulation of insulin. One cup of zucchini has 32% of the RDA for Vitamin C and 2.5 grams of fiber.

Avocado - Avocado is a good source for potassium (twice of what is in bananas) and Vitamin E. Its raw fat (omega 9) content helps the body absorb fat soluble nutrients in other foods eaten in conjunction. A 2005 study showed that eating avocado with a meal helped the body absorb three to five times more carotenoids antioxidant molecules, which protects against free radical damages.

Extra virgin olive oil – Although native to the Mediterranean basin, wild olives were collected as far back as the eighth millennium BC. Omega 9 fatty acids are mono unsaturated fats that have anti-inflammatory properties to them. It assists with less oxidation of LDLs as well as balances fatty acids in the body.

Cilantro – Besides being a great addition to flavor many Hispanic, Asian and Middle Eastern dishes, cilantro has strong antioxidant properties to it. In addition, it has been used as a tea to assist with stomach discomfort. Cilantro is one of the richest herbal sources of Vitamin K and quercetin. The herb is also a good source of calcium, potassium and iron.

Plum – Plums are rich in dietary fiber, assisting with digestion and constipation. They are rich in lutein and zeaxanthin – anti oxidant agents the scavenge free radicals. Zeaxanthin is a carotenoid that is selectively absorbed into the retina for eye heath. Plums are rich in potassium, important for fluid regulation in the body.

Bell peppers – Colored bell peppers, especially red, are rich in vitamin A, which helps in fighting off infections. The Vitamin C, lutein and zeaxanthin help protect the eyes as well as boost the immune function. Only two foods carry two-thirds of all these nutrients - vitamin C, vitamin E, and six of these carotenoids alpha-carotene, beta-carotene, lycopene, lutein, cryptoxanthin and zeaxanthin – tomatoes and sweet bell peppers, as well as containing health supportive sulphur (like garlic and onions do).

Apples – Apples are known for their health benefits and here is why. Their high flavonoid and Vitamin C levels are two properties known to keep the immune system strong. Their high fiber content assists with slow digestion to keep sugar levels steady. They also contain quercetin that has anti-cancer properties to it.

Lemon – Lemons are full of Vitamin C, flavonoids and potassium. Ancient Egyptians believed eating lemons and drinking their juice was effective protection against various poisons. Research has shown lemon balm has a calming effect and inhaling lemon oil increases concentration and alertness.

Pear – The ancient Chinese used pears to treat stomach and lung disorders. One medium pear contains 5.5 grams of fiber, which is needed to absorb vitamins and minerals from your food as well as avoid constipation and, in turn, keep you from developing hemorrhoids.

Carrot - Carrots are rich in poly-acetylene antioxidant falcarinol. Research study conducted by scientists at University of Newcastle on laboratory animals has found that falcarinol in carrots may help fight against cancers by destroying pre-cancerous cells in the tumors. They also compose healthy levels of minerals like copper, calcium, potassium, manganese and phosphorus. Potassium is an important component of cell and body fluids that helps controlling heart rate and blood pressure by countering effects of sodium.

Walnut - A walnut a day may keep bad cholesterol away, according to a 2010 study in the Archives of Internal Medicine that found a 7.4 percent reduction in "bad" LDL cholesterol and an 8.3 percent reduction in the ratio of LDL to HDL, reported WebMD. What's more, triglyceride concentrations declined by more than 10 percent. Brazil nuts, walnuts and cashews can all play a role in reducing the risk of heart disease, according to a Harvard review. Walnuts supply the body with a hefty shot of the amino acid L-ARGININE. It's converted to nitric oxide, a compound that causes blood vessels to dilate, improving the blood flow to all your muscles.

Mint - Dried peppermint leaves have even been found in several Egyptian pyramids carbon dating back to 1,000 BC. The menthol oil derived from mint can be very soothing for nausea and related motion sickness. The aroma of mint activates the salivary glands in our mouth as well as glands which secrete digestive enzymes, thereby facilitating digestion.

Ginger - The University of Maryland Medical Center writes that ginger has been used in China for over 2,000 years to help digestion and treat diarrhea, nausea and stomach upsets. A study published in the November 2003 issue of *Life Sciences* suggests that at least one reason for ginger›s beneficial effects is the free radical protection afforded by one of its active phenolic constituents, 6-gingerol. For nausea, ginger tea made by steeping one or two half-inch slices (one 1/2-inch slice equals 2/3 of an ounce) of fresh ginger in a cup of hot water will likely be all you need to settle your stomach.

Cucumber - Cucumbers are now known to contain lariciresinol, pinoresinol, and secoisolariciresinol—three lignans that have a strong history of research in connection with reduced risk of cardiovascular disease as well as several cancer types, including breast, uterine, ovarian, and prostate cancers. Cucumbers are a rich source of triterpene phytonutrients called cucurbitacins. Cucurbitacins A, B, C, D, and E are all contained in fresh cucumber. They have been the subject of active and ongoing research to determine the extent and nature of their anti-cancer properties. Scientists have already determined that several different signaling pathways (for example, the JAK-STAT and MAPK pathways) required for cancer cell development and survival can be blocked by activity of cucurbitacins. We expect to see human studies that confirm the anti-cancer benefits of cucumbers in the everyday diet.

Swiss Chard - Chard leaves contain at least thirteen different polyphenol antioxidants, including kaempferol, the cardioprotective flavonoid that's also found in broccoli, kale, strawberries, and other foods. But alongside of kaempferol, one of the primary flavonoids found in the leaves of chard is a flavonoid called syringic acid. Syringic acid has received special attention in recent research due to its blood sugar regulating properties. Betalain pigments in chard have been shown to provide antioxidant, anti-inflammatory, and detoxification support.

Peach - Peaches are native to China, from where they spread to rest of the world via ancient silk route. They are rich in many vital minerals such as potassium, fluoride and iron. Iron is required for red blood cell formation. Peaches contain health-promoting flavonoid poly phenolic antioxidants such as *lutein, zea-xanthin* and *ß-cryptoxanthin*. These compounds help act as protective scavengers against oxygen-derived free radicals and reactive oxygen species (ROS) that play a role in aging and various disease processes.

Blueberries - Blueberries are high in manganese, which plays an important role in bone development. One cup of raw blueberries contains four grams of fiber, or over fifteen percent of the recommended daily intake. The soluble fiber present in blueberries can absorb ten to fifteen times its own weight in water, drawing fluid into your gut and increasing bowel movements. New studies make it clear that we can freeze blueberries without doing damage to their delicate anthocyanin antioxidants.

Sunflower seeds - The seeds are especially rich in poly-unsaturated fatty acid *linoleic acid*, which comprise more 50% fatty acids in them. They are also good in mono-unsaturated *oleic acid* that helps **lower LDL** or "bad cholesterol" and increases HDL or "good-cholesterol" in the blood. Sunflower seeds are indeed a very rich source of **vitamin E**; contain about 35.17 g per100 g (about 234% of RDA). Vitamin E is a powerful lipid soluble antioxidant, required for maintaining the integrity of cell membrane of mucus membranes and skin by protecting it from harmful oxygen-free radicals. Sunflower seeds contain health benefiting poly-phenol compounds such as **chlorogenic acid, quinic acid,** and **caffeic acids.** These are natural anti-oxidants, which help remove harmful oxidant molecules from the body. Further, chlorogenic acid helps reduce blood sugar levels by limiting glycogen breakdown in the liver.

Pine nuts - Pine nuts have long made up a part of the American diet; they were staple foods in many Native American cultures. They were eaten as far back as 10,000 years ago, according to Michelle Hansen at the University of Oregon. Pine nuts provide generous amounts of the essential vitamins E and K. Vitamin K allows you to form clots to prevent bleeding after injury; while vitamin E helps you produce red blood cells essential for oxygen transport. They are also rich in manganese, iron, magnesium and zinc.

Cashews - Magnesium in cashews helps in making the bones strong. It helps in providing the right posture of the bone structure for the body. Magnesium prevents the entry of calcium into the nerve cells, thus providing proper functioning of the nervous system. It contains a flavonoid called proanthocyanidins, which inhibits the development of tumor and prevents the growth of cancer cells. Cashew is helpful in combating diabetes as cashew seed extracts helps in restricting the absorption of glucose in the body.

Cauliflower – It's full of vitamin C, a proven antioxidant that boosts immunity and protects against cancer. It's also an excellent, low-calorie source of potassium, says New York City nutritionist Stephanie Middleberg, R.D. Cauliflower also offers fiber and folic acid and contains a sulfur compound called isothiocyanate that protects health and prevents disease.

Mango - Mangos have been used for centuries as medicine and food. The mango fruit contains vitamins A, C and D along with beta-carotene. Vitamin A benefits the body by promoting the health of the skin, immune system and eyes and by supporting cell differentiation and reproduction. Adequate vitamin A intake may lower your risk of cancer, cataracts and age-related macular degeneration Harvard University Health Services reports that half of a small, peeled mango contains nearly three grams of dietary fiber. Mangoes are rich in both soluble and insoluble fiber. High soluble fiber intake may help prevent elevated blood cholesterol and diabetes, while eating plenty of insoluble fiber can regulate bowel movements.

Lime - Lime has an irresistible scent, which causes your mouth to water and this actually aids primary digestion (the digestive saliva floods your mouth even before you taste it). The natural acidity in lime does the rest. While they break down of the macro molecules of the food, the flavonoids, the compounds found in the fragrant oils extracted from lime, stimulate the digestive system and increase secretion of digestive juices, bile and acids. It is a wonderful source of antioxidants & detoxifiers (vitamin-C & flavonoids) which reduce the number of free radicals as well as detoxifying the body.

Basil - The International Herb Society named basil Herb-of-the-Year in 2003. Basil is known to have strong antioxidant properties, especially the extract or oil. Research has established that basil oil contains potent antioxidant, anti-cancer, anti-viral and anti-microbial properties. Many herbalists recommend basil, with its natural antioxidants, to protect the body against damage from free radicals. Antioxidants are an important part of maintaining a healthy diet and lifestyle, and basil may be a safe and effective source of these potent, life-giving compounds (Baritaux et al., 1992).

Dill - During the Middle Ages, people used dill to defend against witchcraft and enchantments. Dill is used for digestion problems including loss of appetite, intestinal gas (flatulence), liver problems, and gallbladder complaints. It is also used for urinary tract disorders including kidney disease and painful or difficult urination. In a study published in "BMC Pharmacology" in 2002, dill weed was also shown to significantly inhibit acid secretion and the development of stomach lesions, providing a level of anti-ulcer activity in laboratory mice.

Fennel - Fennel provides a variety of phytochemicals, including anethole, rutin and quercetin, which function as antioxidants. Antioxidants protect and repair damage resulting from excessive levels of free radicals, chemical byproducts of metabolism. Fennel is a rich source of potassium. Potassium is necessary for a variety of cell, tissue and organ functions. It behaves as an electrolyte, facilitating the conduction of electricity through the body. It also provides the chemicals necessary for muscle contraction utilized in cardiovascular and digestive processes. Their juicy fronds indeed contain several vital vitamins such as pantothenic acid, pyridoxine (vitamin B-6), folic acid, niacin, riboflavin, and thiamin in small but healthy proportions.

Wild Rice - High in fiber and antioxidants, this B complex rich gluten free grain has thirty times greater the antioxidants of white rice and twice as much protein content than brown rice. It is actually a grass, not a grain, that has a high zinc and phosphorous nutrition content known to assist in the immune system.

Cranberries – Cranberries outrank nearly every fruit and vegetable - including strawberries, spinach, broccoli, red grapes, apples, raspberries, and cherries. According to an NBC report, preliminary research from the National Institutes of Health is showing cranberries may prevent tumors form growing rapidly or beginning in the first place.

Northern Beans – Northern beans are the king of fiber with a whopping twelve grams in a cup. They also have 3.77 grams of iron per cup providing 21% of the RDA for iron for women and 47% for men. Supplying 15.2grm protein in a one cup serving, the New England Journal of Medicine 2006 study published "that women who receive the bulk of their protein from vegetable sources like beans may be less likely to develop heart disease"

Garbanzo Beans – These beans are the "happy" beans, rich in B6 to produce serotonin in the body. They are also full of fiber and iron, similar to northern beans. An excellent source of the trace mineral molybdenum, garbanzo beans help in the process of detoxification of sulfites. This mineral is an important component of the enzyme sulfite oxidase, which is involved in this detoxification process.

Coconut Milk - Coconut milk is rich in lauric acid, a medium-chain fatty acid that is abundant in mother's milk. According to the National Center for Biotechnology Information, lauric acid has many germ-fighting, anti-fungal and anti-viral properties that are very effective at ridding the body of viruses, bacteria and countless illnesses. Vitamins C, E and many B vitamins are abundant in coconut milk. Vitamins C and E help to boost the immune system, and B vitamins are responsible for providing energy to the cells. Coconut milk is also rich in magnesium, potassium, phosphorous and iron.

Pumpkin seeds – Pumpkin seeds have a bioavailable source of vitamin E not readily available in food sources. This type of Vitamin E makes pumpkin seeds a great antioxidant to rid the body of free radicals. They are also rich in zinc and magnesium. A quarter-cup of pumpkin seeds has 9.75 grams of protein and 2 grams of fiber. It also contains linoleic acid, and essential fatty acid which the body needs to promote wound healing.

Celery - Celery contains minerals such as calcium, sodium, copper, magnesium, iron, zinc, and potassium. It contains fatty acids and vitamins including vitamin A, C, E, D, B6, B12, and vitamin K. It also contains thiamin, riboflavin, folic acid and fiber. A study at Rutgers University discovered that celery contains anti-cancer compounds that can help stop cancer cells from spreading. One of the components (acetylenics) in celery can actually stop tumor cells from growing. Drinking raw celery juice prevents free-radicals from causing harm to cells and stops the development of cancer in the stomach and the colon.

Pumpkin – Research has shown pumpkin to sow the aging process as well as having a high fiber content to help control blood sugar and bad cholesterol. One cup of cooked pumpkin has 200% of the RDA Vitamin A and has more potassium than a banana.

SUPERFOODS FOR BOOSTING
THE IMMUNE SYSTEM

TURMERIC	COCONUT WATER	GINGER
KIMCHI	SAUERKRAUT	GARLIC
ONIONS	ASPARAGUS	ALL BERRIES
LEMON	CITRUS RIND	POMEGRANATE
CHIA	SEA VEGETABLES	SHIITAKE
MAITAKE	CABBAGE	BRUSSELL SPROUTS
BOK CHOY	CHINESE CABBAGE	BROCCOLI
CAULIFLOWER	LEEKS	SHALLOTS
YAMS	SWEET POTATO	SQUASH
PUMPKIN	APRICOT	BEET
GREEN TEA	QUINOA	AMARANTH
ROSEMARY	THYME	OREGANO
BASIL	MINT	CILANTRO
PUMPKIN SEEDS	ZUCCHINI	ALL BEANS
AVOCADO	PLUM	OILY FISH
OLIVE OIL	COCONUT OIL	SESAME OIL

MORTER ALKALINE FOODS

ALMONDS	GRAPEFRUIT	SWEET POTATOES
APPLES	GRAPES	WHITE POTATOES
APRICOTS	GREEN BEANS	RADISHES
AVOCADOS	GREEN PEAS	RAISINS
BANANAS	LEMONS	RASPBERRIES
DRIED BEANS	LETTUCE	RHUBARB
BEET GREENS	LIMA BEANS	RUTABAGA
BEETS	GREEN LIMA BEANS	SAUERKRAUT
BLACKBERRIES	LIMES	GREEN SOY BEANS
BROCCOLI	GOAT MILK	RAW SPINACH
BRUSSELS SPROUTS	MILLET	STRAWBERRIES
CABBAGE	MOLASSES	TANGERINES
CARROTS	MUSHROOMS	TOMATOES
CAULIFLOWER	ONIONS	WATERCRESS
CELERY	ORANGES	WATERMELON
CHARD LEAVES	PARSNIPS	DRIED FIGS
SOUR CHERRIES	PEACHES	PINEAPPLE
CUCUMBERS	PEARS	DRIED DATES

NATURALLY FERMENTED FOODS

- KIEFER
- SAUERKRAUT
- UMEBOSHI PLUMS

- KOMBUCHA
- SPROUTS
- KIM CHI

MY GO TO SUPPLEMENTS

TOUCHSTONE ESSENTIALS PURE BODY AND SUPERGREENS+D

AVAILABLE AT - https://iamtfw.thegoodinside.com/

ENZYMEDICA DIGEST GOLD AND PRO BIO

BARLEANS FRESH CATCH FISH OILS

FOOD ANTAGONISTS TO AVOID

- GLUTEN - WHEAT, BARLEY, OAT, KAMUT, RYE, SPELT
- CORN
- SOY
- SUGAR
- DAIRY
- MSG
- DISODIUM INOSINATE
- DISODIUM GUANYLATE
- ALL ARTIFICIAL SWEETENERS
- POTATO TOMATO PEPPERS EGGPLANT TOBACCO

TASTY GLUTEN FREE BRANDS

PAMELA'S (BAKED GOODS AND MIXES)

TINKAYADA (PASTA)

GLUTEN FREE PANTRY (BAKE MIXES)

AMY'S (PREPARED FOODS, MUST READ LABELS FOR GLUTEN AND VEGAN PRODUCTS)

ARROWHEAD MILLS (BAKE MIXES, READ LABELS FOR GLUTEN FREE CHOICES)

GLUTINO (WAFER AND SANDWICH COOKIES)

IAN'S (READ FOR GLUTEN FREE CHOICES, BAKE MIXES AND CHICKEN TENDERS)

BELL AND EVAN'S (READ FOR GLUTEN FREE OPTIONS, CHICKEN TENDERS)

UDI'S (BREAD, MUFFINS)

RUDI'S (BREAD, READ FOR GLUTEN FREE CHOICES)

VAN'S (WAFFLES, PANCAKES AND FRENCH TOAST, READ LABEL COMPLETELY FOR GLUTEN FREE OPTIONS)

DAIRY FREE OPTIONS

(Goat and Sheep milk still contains casein)

GOAT CHEESE

SHEEP CHEESE

SO DELICIOUS COCONUT ICE CREAM AND BARS (READ LABELS FOR COCONUT VS. SOY)

COCONUT BLISS ICE CREAM

RICE DREAM ICE CREAM BARS (NOT SO MUCH THE ICE CREAM)

ENDANGERED SPECIES DARK CHOCOLATE

EARTH BALANCE BUTTER

ALMOND MILK, UNSWEETENED ORIGINAL FOR COOKING

ALMOND MILK, UNSWEETENED VANILLA FOR DRINKING

COFFEE OPTIONS

YERBA MATE

GREEN TEA

WHITE TEA

RECOMMENDED READING

Pain Free Living: The Egoscue Method for Strength, Harmony, and Happiness, Pete Egoscue

The Cheat System Diet, Jackie Wicks

Stress Less (for Women): Calm Your Body, Slow Aging, and Rejuvenate the Mind in 5 Simple Steps, Thea Singer

Eat Right 4 Your Blood Type series, Peter J. D'Adamo

The Sonoma Diet: Trimmer Waist, Better Health in Just 10 Days!, Connie Guttersen and Stephanie Karpinske

Anti-Cancer a New Way of Life, David Servn-Schreiber

The Raw Food Detox Diet: The Five-Step Plan for Vibrant Health and Maximum Weight Loss, Natalia Rose

The Whole 30, Melissa Hartwig and Dallas Hartwig

All In: You Are One Decision Away From a Totally Different Life, Mark Batterson

What to Eat If You Have Cancer, Maureen Keane, M. A.

Grain Brain: The Surprising Truth about Wheat, Carbs, and Sugar—Your Brain's Silent Killers, David Perlmutter

The Power of Habit: Why We Do What We Do in Life and Business, Charles Duhigg

Foods to Fight Cancer, Richard Beliveau, P. A.

The Cancer Survivor's Guide, Neal Barnard, M. A.,

The Power of Positive Thinking Trilogy, Norman Vincent Peale

Works Cited

Ballentine, R. M. (2007). *Diet & Nutrition A Holistic Approach.* USA: Himalayan Institute Press.

David Servn-Schreiber, M. (2008). *Anti Cancer a New Way of Life.*

Hoffer, A. M. (1978). *Putting it All Together: The New Orthomolecular Nutrition.* New Canaan: Keats Publishing, Inc.

Lepore, D. N. (1985). *Ultimate Healing System: The Illustrated Guide to Muscle Testing & Nutrition.* Jersey City: Don Lepore.

Loomis Jr., H. F. (2007). *Enzymes The Key to Health Vol. 1 The Fundamentals.* Madison: 21st Century Nutrition Publishing.

Maureen Keane, M. A., and Daniella, Chace. M.S, (2007). *What to Eat If You Have Cancer.*

Morter Jr., M. T. (2009). *Your Health... Your Choice...* Hollywood: Frederick Fell Publishers, Inc.

Neal Barnard, Md., and Jenifer K Reilly, Rd., (2008). *The Cancer Survivor's Guide.*

Richard Beliveau, P. a. (2007). *Foods to Fight Cancer.*

Mercola.Com

Huffingtonpost.Com

Mensfitness.Com

Livestrong.Com

Webmd.Com

Nbcnews.Com

Whfoods.Com

Nutritionandyou.Com

Greenmedinfo.Com

Voices.Yahoo.Com

Yournutritiouschoices.Com

Beliefnet.Com Wikipedia.Org

Healhtyeating.Sfgate.Com

Citrus.Com

Acknowledgements

THANK YOU

37 years in the making (17 years in hospitality, 20 years in health food stores and private chefing), The Real Language of Food is the culmination of what you are cooking. Where do I begin?

Thank you, God, for having me realize that everything falls into place at the right time. This book has been ready to be published for 3 years, and it is at this time, right now, that I am thankful that it had to wait.

My parents, RIP, Salvatore and Dolly Falcone, you encouraged us since babies to be all we could be and that we could go beyond the moon and the stars. Cooking show is next Mama and Papa.

Thank you, Jeff Godsell, my husband. Receiving a TBI 8 years ago really changed the course of our family's life and you have been supportive with all the modifications that we have had to make to keep our fast-paced life going with 3 children. On the course of modifying our lives, is how this book came into play. Better nutrition has really made my healing so much more enhanced, and realizing even more so then, how important it was to reach mass amounts of people on food and health both total body and brain function. Thank you, my love, for helping me be me on this journey of healing and our life together.

Thank you to our children, Lexi, Maxim and Quentin,

who gave me the WHY I need to stay on my health journey to be the healthiest possible me.

Thank you, April and Mike Voukon, through college and beyond, a truer support system one cannot find.

Julie Ann Whitley Green, your belief and faith in me never ending.

Maria Elena And Craig D'Amico, my sis and bro in law. As opposite as we are, greater back up in family life as only you guys can give.

Pete Egoscue, Brian Bradley, Christi Slaven, and Michael Bellofatto for providing me with the ability to share Pain Free Living and empower those who think they are not be able to strengthen and tone for their optimal health.

Dawn Langnes Shear, Chief Development Officer, Upledger Institute International and Barral Institute International for having the privilege of cooking for you and speaking the Real Language of Food.

Andrew Giordano D.C., who knew this is where we would end up, lol.

Jill Smith – my first health food friend that I connected with.

Stephanie Crank, Pilates Movement Studio, truly an inspiration in my life and a bright light. You are the embodiment of strength and grace.

Erin Connor, Personal Trainer, who knew that a LinkedIn contact would end up being such a sister in arms? Thank you for being such a stronghold in my life.

Sarah Bingham LDN, Fast Food Healing, my Nutrition Twinsie.

Jill Federici, the newest in my tribe, thank you for all the last-minute challenges to keep me on my toes.

Michelle Chandler, not sure I would be here without you.

Nature's Finest Foods (which is now Earth Origins) – Pam and Moses Brown and Judy Veal, Abby's Health and Nutrition – Abby Sayler, and Chuck's Natural Foods – Chuck Homuth. In this order, this is where my culinary health adventures began, and I was able to cultivate and hone my health food skills, taking in as much knowledge and training to mesh food and health together.

Wendy Cheatham, "I am" are the strongest words our Lord gave us.

Dr. John Camp, USF Head of Liberal Studies. It is because of him accepting me into the liberal studies program that I fell back into my culinary dream in 1988.

Chef Ann Leighton, you taught me my future was in my hands and no one else's.

Jerry Hudgens, "Just let her get a taste of it and she's off and running!"

Chef Ed Valenti, for encouraging me to spread my wings and fly.

Jessica Hope, Brain Injured Blondes take on the World. I have come so far because of you, your love, and your support.

Cheryl Bartlett Schuette LMT, Advanced Massage and Colon Hydrotherapy, are we doing another Sprint Tri next year together?

The Root Cause Clinic and Staff

Laura Muchmore, for having me be your Foodie Consultant.

Brandi Stewart microscopist Stewart Analysis live blood cell analysis

Suzanne Grey, colon hydrotherapist ReNew Life Wellness

Mari Velar for being my silent assistant, sounding board and cheerleader through this.

Amy Rinkevich, RN who fine-tuned my last ¼ mile.

Joanne Muir, Shaman, LMT, you were there at this book's conception.

Dr. Kristen Carla, D.O.M., NCCAOM, getting my balance back in record time.

Sherry Bell Life Management Center.

Elisa Di Falco MLD Institute International

Ann Witt, LMHC Piewise Living and Kai Chi Do instructor – all must try Kai Chi Do to know what I am talking about.

Rosie Charles, PRP Wine, you are better than the finest wine.

All my clients over the years that have given me culinary challenges in striving to be a better chef.

Eli Gonzalez , Lil Barcaski and TGP for making this

dream readable, Lol.

All my colleagues and friends I may have missed – I love you all.

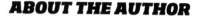

ABOUT THE AUTHOR

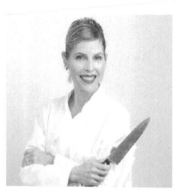

Holistic Chef Adrienne Falcone Godsell, B.A. Liberal Studies USF, Tampa, Fl., A.S. Culinary Arts Johnson and Wales University, N. Miami, Fl., began her adventures in the culinary field at fourteen, when her parents opened a traditional Italian deli/ catering business in Fort Myers, Florida. That little nibble of the hospitality industry had her hooked, taking her on a journey of kitchens that include Moffit Cancer Center Tampa, Fl.; Kamaaina award winning restaurant Horatio's Honolulu, Hi; Registry Resort Naples, FL; opening Seattle restaurant Palisade; Don CeSar Maritana Grille, St. Pete Beach, Fl; and then fell into the world of natural foods in 1998. It was there that she finally found her culinary calling, taking her years of experience and plugged it in to the world of 'Food For Health.' Adrienne has taken 'health food' to new heights, always searching for ways to make healthy eating practical and affordable. As a working mother of three, she knows the challenges of eating healthy and making it flavorful without making a huge mess in the kitchen ('we don't get the luxury of having dishwashers at home the way we do in the industry').

Adrienne applies the same work ethics she uses in her home kitchen that she uses in the field – cost effective, non-labor-intensive recipes – to keep her and her own family going as well as her personal chef profession.

Adrienne wants to Share the Health with everyone, via Skype or in-home cooking lessons; cooking classes, dinner parties and wine pairings and corporate lunch and learns.

Adrienne can be reached at email
afalconegodsell@gmail.com

813-990-7428

Instagram@iamthefoodwhisperer

LinkedIn Adrienne Falcone Godsell

As heard on

Joel Chudnow's **Hawk Health Hour – Hawk Radio**

Brandon Rimes' **Real Estate Quarterback Radio Show 1380 AM Tampa Bay**

Sarah Bingham's **Snot Nosed Kids Podcast**

Testimonials

Adrienne was a delight to work with on my health and nutrition! For years, I suffered from stomach issues - I was even hospitalized twice for the severe pain. I took many tests - even had an endoscopy - and every GI doctor I visited told me it was irritable bowel. I did not see much improvement with their suggestions. Then I consulted with Adrienne. She put me on a nutrition plan and probiotics, and within weeks, I was feeling better physically and emotionally. Adrienne was able to help me identify what foods were triggering negative reactions and which foods I could use to replace them. She even cooked meals for me and taught me how to make delicious nutritious foods that would agree with my stomach. I learned a lot about foods and nutrition and most importantly, I learned how to manage my health issues. Adrienne was invaluable to my health!

Julie Avila Stuckman
Marketing and Advertising Professional

* * *

Adrienne came to my rescue when food sensitivities required me to adopt an entirely different way of eating. She took me food shopping, making great suggestions of how to substitute or avoid the offending ingredients, and created my own personal set of recipes for me!

Jill B. Independent
Sr. Sales Director

* * *

My boyfriend felt the need to learn how to cook fish and shrimp as he had no idea how to season it or cook it. We hired Adrienne to come to our home and give him a 2hr class. He learned several ways to season several kinds of fish and several ways to make it. As a bonus, Adrienne taught him how to make a reduction sauce from scratch using shrimp. My bf is super excited. He learned how to mince garlic and after Adrienne left, he said he feels more confident in the kitchen and more creative. Adrienne is AMAZINGLY knowledgeable in cooking healthy for ANY type of "diet" or restriction and she can adjust the recipe to meet those dietary needs. She is a wealth of knowledge in nutrition and we are truly appreciative of what she taught us in a nonjudgmental way. I would definitely recommend Adrienne for ANY cooking class needs as well as healthy cooking services.

NCEA Certified Master Aesthetician, Health Educator and Yoga Instructor

* * *

Before I started eating Adrienne's food I had been having a lot of stomach and skin issues. When I would eat certain things I would break out in hives, or just not feel great afterwards. Once I started eating the food she was making me, I really started to notice a difference. I have not broken out in hives once since I've been eating her way. I noticed a lot of the health issues I had been having before were no longer a problem. I no longer had heartburn after my meals, and I didn't have that bloated shouldn't have eaten that feeling either. Eating her food has also helped a lot with that after lunch lull that I always felt, and I was able to continue to focus throughout the day! Over all it was an adjustment as I love fast food, carbs and anything else that probably isn't good for you. However, once I realized how much better I was feeling, it would be hard to go back to just eating whatever. Thank you Adrienne, for making great food, and being one of my cheerleaders during this experience.

Anna, sales